REGULATION
of HAEMOGLOBIN
SYNTHESIS

REGULATION
of HAEMOGLOBIN
SYNTHESIS

J. NEUWIRT, M. D. and P. POŇKA, M. D.

Department of Pathological Physiology,
Faculty of Medicine,
Charles University, Prague

1977

MARTINUS NIJHOFF / MEDICAL DIVISION
THE HAGUE

ISBN 90.247.1999.2

Copyright 1977 by Martinus Nijhoff, Publishers, P.O. Box 269, The Hague, The Netherlands

© Translation: K. Ošancová, M.D.

This book is published with the arrangement of

AVICENUM, Czechoslovak Medical Press, Prague

Printed in Czechoslovakia

CONTENTS

ABBREVIATIONS 8
ACKNOWLEDGEMENT 9

1. INTRODUCTION 11

2. SUBSTRATE SUPPLY FOR HAEMOGLOBIN SYNTHESIS 14

IRON UPTAKE 14
  Mechanism of iron supply to erythroid cells 15
  Factors influencing iron uptake by erythroid cells 20
    Iron and transferrin levels and transferrin saturation 20
    Metabolic state of erythroid cells 21
    The role of sulfhydryl groups in iron uptake 22
    Other factors which influence iron uptake 23
    Iron uptake from chelating agents 23
  Intracellular kinetics of iron 24
    Ferritin 25
    Other non-haem iron proteins and iron complexes 26
    Mitochondrial iron 27
    Inhibitors of haem synthesis as a tool in investigations of the intracellular kinetics
     of iron 28
  Regulation of iron supply for haemoglobin synthesis 34
    Effect of haem on iron uptake by reticulocytes 36
    Effect of inhibitors of haem and globin syntheses on iron uptake 38
    Mechanism of the effect of haem on iron uptake 45
REGULATION OF UPTAKE OF GLYCINE AND OTHER AMINO ACIDS 50

3. HAEM SYNTHESIS 55

BIOSYNTHESIS OF HAEM 55
  General introduction 55
  ALA synthesis 59
  ALA synthetase 61
  Porphobilinogen (PBG) synthesis. ALA dehydrase enzyme 64
  Conversion of porphobilinogen (PBG) to uroporphyrinogen III 64
  Conversion of uroporphyrinogen to coproporphyrinogen by the enzyme uroporphyri-
   nogen decarboxylase 66

Conversion of coproporphyrinogen to protoporphyrinogen by the enzyme coproporphyrinogen oxidase 66
Combination of iron with protoporphyrin 66
Free protoporphyrin 68
REGULATION OF HAEM BIOSYNTHESIS 69
Enzyme synthesis 70
Changes in enzyme activity 74
Regulation by substrate supply 82
Metabolic and external factors 84
Haem catabolism 85

4. GLOBIN SYNTHESIS 87

GLOBIN BIOSYNTHESIS 87
General introduction 87
Role of ribonucleic acids in globin synthesis 89
Messenger RNA 89
Isolation and identification of globin mRNA 90
Methods used for the isolation of globin mRNA 91
Detection of messenger RNA for globin 95
Characteristics of globin mRNA 100
Biosynthesis of globin mRNA 104
Transfer RNA 106
Ribosomes and globin synthesis 107
Ribosome structure 107
The role of polyribosomes 110
The role of sub-units 111
Membrane-bound ribosomes 112
Function of the active ribosomal complex 112
Initiation of the globin chain 113
Initiation of globin synthesis by means of methionyl-tRNA 113
Initiation factors of reticulocyte ribosomes 117
Elongation of the globin chain 119
Globin chain termination 121
REGULATION OF GLOBIN SYNTHESIS 122
Post-transcription control of globin synthesis 124
Stability of globin mRNA 124
Translation control 125
Rate limiting step in the synthesis of the globin chain 126
Synchronization of synthesis of different chains 127
The role of haem in globin synthesis 129

5. REGULATION OF HAEMOGLOBIN SYNTHESIS 135

COORDINATION OF HAEM AND GLOBIN SYNTHESES 135
Regulatory role of haem 136

Mutual relations between haem and globin syntheses 139
HAEMOGLOBIN SYNTHESIS DURING MATURATION 144

6. DIFFERENTIATION OF ERYTHROID CELLS 149

ERYTHROID DIFFERENTIATION IN HAEMATOPOIETIC TISSUE AND
THE INITIATION OF HAEMOGLOBIN SYNTHESIS 150
Mechanism of erythropoietin action 151
ERYTHROID DIFFERENTIATION WITHOUT ERYTHROPOIETIN 158

7. ANAEMIAS DUE TO DISORDERS OF HAEMOGLOBINIZATION 161

HYPOCHROMIC ANAEMIAS DUE TO IMPAIRED HAEM SYNTHESIS 163
Hypochromic anaemias caused by a reduced iron supply into erythroid tissue 163
Iron deficiency anaemia 163
Congenital atransferrinaemia 166
Hypochromic anaemia as a result of reduced iron release from reticuloendothelial
cells 167
Copper defficiency 167
Sideroblastic anaemias 167
HYPOCHROMIC ANAEMIAS DUE TO IMPAIRED GLOBIN SYNTHESIS 172
Thalassaemia 172
α-thalassaemia 173
Haemoglobin Constant Spring and related mutants of the terminal portion of the
chain 174
β- and δβ-thalassaemia 176

REFERENCES 174
SUBJECT INDEX 199

ABBREVIATIONS

A	adenylic acid
AIA	allylisopropylacetamide
ALA	δ-aminolaevulinic acid
ATP	adenosine triphosphate
C	cytidylic acid
cAMP	cyclic AMP
cDNA	DNA complementary to RNA
CoA	coenzyme A
dA, dC, dG, dT	the prefix d is added if the sugar of the appropriate nucleotide (A, C, G or T = thymidylic acid) is deoxyribose
DNA	deoxyribonucleic acid
EDTA	ethylenediaminetetraacetate
EF	elongation factors
G	guanylic acid
GTP	guanosine triphosphate
Hb	haemoglobin
HCR	haemin-controlled repressor
HnRNA	heterogeneous nuclear RNA
IF	initiation factors
INH	isonicotinic acid hydrazide
mRNA	messenger RNA
mRNP	messenger ribonucleoprotein
NAD	nicotinamide adenine dinucleotide
NADH	reduced form of NAD
PBG	porphobilinogen
poly (A)	poly (adenylic acid)
RNA	ribonucleic acid
rRNA	ribosomal RNA
tRNA	transfer RNA
U	uridylic acid

ACKNOWLEDGEMENT

We would like to thank our collaborators Dr. J. Borová and Dr. O. Fuchs who helped us with our experimental work. Our thanks are also due to Dr. E. Brdičková who assisted us with the preparation of the literature and finally we wish to thank all technical assistants, H. Stoklasová, A. Gaertnerová and V. Benešová, for the assistance during experimental work and the preparation of the manuscript.

1. INTRODUCTION

Haemoglobin is one of the most important molecules in the animal kingdom. Its function is to carry oxygen to tissues. In lower invertebrates the blood pigment is present in the haemolymph and is not bound in cells. Later in the course of phylogenesis haemoglobin remains associated with cells which produce it and in this form it reaches the peripheral circulation. In higher organisms the haemoglobin production is thus determined by two main factors: haemoglobin synthesis in erythroid cells and the formation of these erythroid cells which depends on cell proliferation in haematopoietic organs.

Human haemoglobin is made up of two chains which combine from four different polypeptide chains formed in varying ratios in different periods of the life cycle. During the life span of humans the following haemoglobins are formed: embryonic haemoglobins Gower 1 and 2, foetal haemoglobin F and two adult haemoglobins A and A_2. ε- and α-chains are part of the embryonic haemoglobins Gower 1 (ε_4) and Gower 2 ($\alpha_2\varepsilon_2$). These haemoglobins predominate in embryos during the second month of pregnancy and at the end of the first trimester they are completely replaced by foetal haemoglobin F ($\alpha_2\gamma_2$). Adult haemoglobin A consists of two α- and two β-chains and is the main component of red cells in adults. A relatively small component of red cells accounting for less than 2% of the total haemoglobin, is haemoglobin A_2 ($\alpha_2\delta_2$). Each of the four polypeptide chains binds one haem group. The molecular weight of the majority of mammalian haemoglobins is between 64,000–69,000 daltons. In addition to the mentioned normal haemoglobins in man, as a result of genetic disturbances, also some pathological haemoglobins may be found. The presence of these haemoglobins may be manifested by enhanced haemolysis, an increased or reduced affinity of haemoglobin for oxygen and by some other disorders.

In man the site of haemoglobin formation changes from the embryonic mesenchyme to the foetal liver and spleen and eventually erythropoiesis is confined to bone marrow.

Haemoglobin is synthesized in special cells of some invertebrates and in erythroid cells of vertebrates. Its synthesis starts in immature erythorid precursors and persists to the stage of reticulocytes. A stimulus for the initiation of haemoglobin synthesis is the action of erythropoietin on unipotent stem cells committed to the erythroid line (so-called erythropoietin-responsive cells). Except for some exceptional circum-

11

stances, as e.g. the action of Friend virus, the presence of erythropoietin is essential for the initiation of haemoglobin synthesis in normal human bone marrow. So far it is not clear by what mechanisms haemoglobin synthesis initiation is controlled in the early embryonic stages.

Similar to all other proteins, globin is synthesized on ribosomes, while mitochondria are the site of haem production. Haem is probably brought by various carriers to ribosomes where it combines with globin and the complete haemoglobin molecule is formed. Iron is delivered to erythroid cells from transferrin and inside the cell it enters into mitochondria.

In general the regulation of haemoglobin formation may be divided into three parts: a) regulation of globin synthesis, b) regulation of haem synthesis and c) regulation of substrate supply, i.e. iron and amino acids. Regulation of globin synthesis is effected at the gene, transcription and post-transcription levels. At the gene level globin synthesis may be influenced by gene duplication or amplification. Regulation of transcription includes regulation of mRNA formation for different globin chains. Finally post-transcription regulation may take place at the level of mRNA processing and includes among other processes the regulation of initiation and elongation of chains and termination of mRNA translation. The availability of different tRNAs and all factors participating in the translation of mRNA is also essential. Regulation at this level also comprises the final formation of the haemoglobin molecule and the formation of tetramers.

The synthesis of porphyrins — the final product being protoporphyrin which combine with iron to form haem — is regulated independently. The key enzyme here is δ-aminolaevulinic acid synthetase and its production is probably affected by a feedback mechanism by haem, the final product of the whole biosynthetic chain. Changes in the activity of this and some other enzymes of the porphyrin chain may also have a certain importance in regulating processes of haem synthesis.

Finally, an important role in haemoglobin synthesis is played by the regulation of the supply of basic building materials — iron and amino acids into erythroid cells.

The haem molecule appears to play a particularly important role in the regulation of haemoglobin synthesis. Haem is not only essential for globin synthesis and renders the formation of tetramers possible but, on the other hand, it also controls its own synthesis by influencing the formation of δ-aminolaevulinic acid synthetase and by regulating the iron uptake by the cell.

The regulation of haemoglobin synthesis is a complex process where the production of individual components of the haemoglobin molecule is very subtly coordinated and only under certain pathological conditions are some of the haemoglobin components produced in reduced amounts or conversely present in the cell in excess. Under such conditions anaemias usually develop which are of considerable importance for clinical haematologists. Iron-deficiency anaemia is one of the most widespread diseases in the world.

The limited size of this monograph did not enable us to discuss some very important aspects of haemoglobin formation. They include e.g. the genetic control of haemoglobin formation, a more detailed analysis of the differentiation in the embryonic period and adult life and finally some clinical problems of anaemias caused by impaired haemoglobinization.

The mechanism of haemoglobin synthesis and its regulation are currently being investigated intensively in many distinguished laboratories in different parts of the world. We tried to summarize in our monograph some of the most important results related to haemoglobin synthesis and to present our small and modest contribution in this field.

2. SUBSTRATE SUPPLY
   FOR HAEMOGLOBIN SYNTHESIS

One of the basic prerequisites for normal haemoglobin synthesis is a regulated supply of substrates to systems producing haem (mitochondria) as well as globin (ribosomes). For the formation of the protein component of haemoglobin all amino acids are essential. On the other hand for the synthesis of the prosthetic group — haem — iron, glycine and succinyl-coenzyme A are needed. Succinyl-coenzyme A is present in non-limiting amounts due to the metabolic activity of mitochondria (see p. 60). While amino acids are available in a free form, iron is bound to its protein carrier — transferrin.

Iron is not only a passive substrate of haem synthesis but also participates in the control of this process. Iron is involved at different enzymatic levels of the haem synthetic pathway and it is assumed that it influences the activity or synthesis of some enzymes. Iron forms part of haem which is essential for globin synthesis. The availability of intracellular iron thus plays an important role in the control of the rate of haemoglobin synthesis. Understanding of mechanisms by which iron enters erythroid cells and the haem molecule is important with regard to haemoglobin synthesis under normal and pathological conditions and therefore considerable attention is paid to them in the present monograph.

IRON UPTAKE

Iron enters all haem synthesizing cells. It is obvious that various cells differ markedly in their capacity to take up iron. Cells of erythropoietic tissue must absorb much more iron than other cells because they produce haemoglobin which requires larger amounts of this metal. Does iron enter erythroid cells in relation to needs for haemoglobin synthesis or is iron uptake regulated separately? It was revealed that iron enters erythroblasts before intensive haemoglobin synthesis begins. However, a certain coordination of both processes — i.e. haemoglobin synthesis and iron uptake by cells — must be assumed because mature erythrocytes contain, under normal conditions, only negligible amounts of non-haem iron. From the subsequent discussion it will ensue that erythroid cells, at least in certain stages, are able to regulate the iron uptake in a definite relation to haemoglobin synthesis.

The close relationship of iron to erythropoiesis is evident from the fact that about 70% of the total iron in the organism are present in the haemoglobin of circulating red cells. This relationship is furthermore supported by ferrokinetic studies which indicate that about 90% of the iron which leaves plasma enters erythroid tissue (*Pollycove*, 1964). Iron metabolism is under normal conditions exceptional because iron moves in a closed circuit (about 90% of iron utilized for haemoglobin synthesis is obtained from aged disintegrated red cells).

In plasma iron is bound reversibly to transferrin. Chemically transferrin is a glyco-protein with a molecular weight of 76,000 daltons (*Feeney* and *Allison*, 1969; *Morgan*, 1974). In electrophoresis it moves like a β_1-globulin and is present in Cohn's fraction IV-7. Every transferrin molecule has two independent binding sites which can bind two iron atoms. Iron (ferric iron) is at a normal pH and P_{CO_2} extremely firmly bound to transferrin and the apparent equilibrium constant for the reaction between trans-ferrin and iron is approximately $10^{24} M^{-1}$ (*Aasa et al.*, 1963; *Aisen* and *Leibman*, 1968). Spontaneous iron dissociation is therefore impossible and in cells which are able to take up iron from transferrin there a special mechanism for release of iron from the binding protein must exist (*see* p. 22). At each binding site in the binding of Fe^{3+} three tyrosyl residues and two imidazole residues are involved (*Komatsu* and *Feeney*, 1967). During binding of every iron atom to transferrin three hydrogen ions are released from the protein and simultaneously one bicarbonate ion is added (for reference *see Bezkorovainy* and *Zschocke*, 1974; *Morgan*, 1974). Bicarbonate can be replaced by another ion (e.g. oxalate or malonate) but then the ability to release iron from the transferrin−iron−anion complex to erythroid cells deteriorates markedly (*Aisen* and *Leibman*, 1973). It cannot even be ruled out that carbonate and not bicarbonate is the sixth ligande in the iron−transferrin complex (*Bates* and *Schlabach*, 1973, 1975). It has been suggested that the carbonate ion interacts with positive charges on the protein via two of its oxygens and that it donates a co-ordinate bond to Fe^{3+} via the third oxygen.

MECHANISM OF IRON SUPPLY TO ERYTHROID CELLS

In 1957 *Bessis* and *Breton-Gorius* (*see Bessis*, 1963) elaborated a theory, based on electron microscopic studies, that iron in red blood cells originates from the ferritin of reticulum cells. Their electron micrographs show erythroblasts forming small islands in the bone marrow round large reticuloendothelial cells and the authors suggested the functional importance of these anatomical units. At the site of contact between the reticulum cell and cytoplasm of the erythroblast on the surface of the latter small invaginations develop which become closed and form small vacuoles which penetrate into the cytoplasm of the erythroblast. This phenomenon related to pinocytosis was described by *Policard* and *Bessis* as ropheocytosis. By means of ropheocytosis erythroblasts incorporate particles of the cytoplasm of the central reticuloendothelial cell (nurse cell) which normally contains numerous ferritin mole-cules.

The research of many other scientists calls, however, for a critical evaluation of the hypothesis expressed by *Bessis et al.* Some workers suggested the possibility that part of the ferritin may migrate from erythroblasts to the reticular cell. Moreover, as emphasized by *Bessis* and *Breton-Gorius* (1962), it is very difficult to estimate the quantitative importance of ropheocytosis for iron supply to erythroid precursors. Ferrokinetic investigations indicate (*Pollycove* and *Mortimer*, 1961; *Hosain* and *Finch*, 1964; *Najean et al.*, 1967) that almost all iron utilized for haemoglobin synthesis passes through plasma. *Lajtha* and *Suit* (1955) showed that only immature red cells take up significant amounts of radioiron bound to transferrin. Direct transfer from reticular cells and bypassing of plasma is obviously insignificant, as compared with iron transport from plasma into maturing red cells.

Some morphological studies also give no support to *Bessis'* hypothesis. *Jones* (1964, 1965) observed pinocytosis on the membrane of young erythroblasts but did not find any evidence of the functional importance of erythroblastic islets. It is possible that this pinocytic activity does not reflect the ferritin uptake but that it is associated with the transferrin uptake by erythroblasts (*Appleton et al.*, 1971). The observations of *Tanaka et al.* (1966) do not support the hypothesis that ferritin is shifted directly from the reticulum cell into the adjacent erythroblast. These authors assume that ferritin in erythroid precursors originates from iron brought to the cell membrane by means of transferrin and from ferritin which is synthesized on this membrane.

On the other hand, it is important to mention that erythroblasts are able to take up ferritin *in vitro* and to expel it again (*Tanaka*, 1970). The electronmicroscopic picture of the expulsion process differs, however, markedly from ropheocytosis.

Today it is generally accepted that ferritin taken up by pinocytosis cannot play an important role as a source of iron for haemoglobin synthesis. The majority of workers support the view that erythropoietic cells obtain iron directly from transferrin (*Walsh et al.*, 1949; *Jandl et al.*, 1959). Immature erythroid cells, in the same way as mature erythrocytes, may take up transferrin-free iron, but iron which is not bound to transferrin is, however, poorly utilized for haem synthesis. Very important evidence of the specific role of transferrin as a source of iron for erythroid tissue is provided by the clinical picture in congenital atransferrinaemia (*Heilmayer et al.*, 1961; *Čáp et al.*, 1968; *Goya et al.*, 1972). In all patients severe hypochromic anaemia and generalized siderosis was described. The virtue of transferrin thus lies not only in iron transport in plasma but also in its ability to release iron to cells according to their requirements.

The main source of iron for its incorporation into cells which produce haemoglobin is thus **transferrin.** It is, however, possible that serum contains other factors than transferrin which facilitate iron incorporation into erythroid cell precursors (*Najean et al.*, 1960; *Najean*, 1961; *Workman et al.*, 1975). *Eldor et al.* (1970) did not observe that iron incorporation into reticulocytes was stimulated by transferrin-free serum but they described that in the presence of normal human serum, incorporated iron is more readily utilized for haem synthesis.

The transfer of iron from transferrin into erythroid cells was studied in detail mainly using reticulocytes incubated with plasma or purified transferrin. For labelling ^{59}Fe is used, less frequently ^{55}Fe. The protein component of transferrin can be labelled with ^{125}I or ^{131}I.

Detailed investigations of *Morgan* and *Laurell* (1963), *Morgan* (1964) and *Baker* and *Morgan* (1969a, 1971) revealed that for the transfer of iron into reticulocytes a reversible transferrin uptake by cells is necessary. Transferrin uptake takes place in three stages. The first stage is independent of temperature and is insensitive to metabolic inhibitors. This immediate transferrin uptake represents adsorption of transferrin on the erythroid cell surface.

During the subsequent $10-15$ min of incubation at $37\,^{\circ}C$ the amount of transferrin in erythroid cells increases progressively. This stage depends on the temperature and is maximal at a physiological pH and ionic strength and is inhibited by certain metabolic inhibitors, mainly sulfhydryl reacting agents. It seems that this phase involves the development of a stronger union between reticulocyte and transferrin (*Morgan*, 1964; *Baker* and *Morgan*, 1971; *Morgan*, 1974).

After about 15min incubation a dynamic equilibrium is established between transferrin molecules in the medium and on reticulocytes and the amount of labelled transferrin in cells does not increase further during subsequent reticulocyte incubation. On the other hand, iron uptake continues with increasing time of incubation. This finding can be explained by the fact that transferrin released back into the medium after giving up iron to reticulocytes is replaced by other transferrin molecules with iron (*Jandl* and *Katz*, 1963; *Morgan* and *Laurell*, 1963).

In the stage of initial adsorption of transferrin on cell, transferrin reacts with specific binding sites or receptors on the cell membrane (*Jandl et al.*, 1959, *Katz*, 1965, 1970; *Morgan*, 1974). Recently several groups of authors were able to solubilize — by means of detergents — transferrin from reticulocyte stroma in the form of a complex with a membrane component. This membrane component is most probably a transferrin receptor (*Garret et al.*, 1973; *Speyer* and *Fielding*, 1974; *Fielding* and *Speyer*, 1974; *van Bockxmeer et al.*, 1975; *Sly et al.*, 1975b). The molecular weight of the protein receptor is about 150,000 daltons and some evidence was provided that it is made up of two sub-units.

Originally it was assumed that iron is released from transferrin which remains bound to membrane receptors of immature erythroid cells (*Jandl* and *Katz*, 1963; *Katz*, 1965, 1970). *Morgan* and *Appleton* (1969), however, provided later evidence that another probable way exists by which erythroid cells obtain iron from transferrin. These authors assume, on the basis of their studies, that the whole transferrin molecule carrying iron, penetrates into the intracellular space of the reticulocyte. After incubation of the reticulocytes with transferrin labelled with ^{125}I it is possible to

17

detect the isotope in the cytoplasm of reticulocytes by electron microscopic autoradiography (*Morgan* and *Appleton*, 1969). The authors made numerous control experiments which provided evidence that the method used is suited for locating transferrin molecules inside the cell. They demonstrated that inside the cells there is much more transferrin-^{125}I when the incubation takes place at 37°C that at 4°C. They also ruled out the possibility that ^{125}I could be released from transferrin and only mimic labelled transferrin in the cell. In their subsequent investigation, *Appleton, Morgan* and *Baker* (1971) tried to visualize the movement of transferrin by conjugating the transferrin with ferritin which can be detected by electron microscopy. After incubation of reticulocytes with the conjugate of ferritin and transferrin, the conjugate was observed particularly in invaginations on the surface of reticulocytes and in intracellular vesicles (Fig. 1). It thus seems that transferrin penetrates through the reticulocyte membrane by endocytosis. Many agents which inhibit the function of microtubules (colchicin, vinblastine, vincristine, strychnine, heavy water) reduce the transferrin uptake and thus also the iron uptake by reticulocytes and bone-marrow cells. These results suggest that in the process of transferrin penetration into erythroid cells microtubular-like proteins are involved (*Hemmaplardh et al.*, 1974).

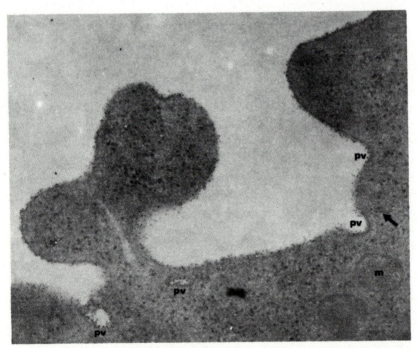

Fig. 1. Electronmicrograph of reticulocyte incubated with ferritin-conjugated trasferrin. Conjugated ferritin is located on membranes and in pinocytotic vesicles (p.v.) shown in various stages of formation. Arrow shows free conjugated ferritin in the cytoplasm. (From *Appleton et al.*, 1971. Reproduced with the permission of the authors.)

As some workers still doubt that transferrin passes through the outer cell membrane into the interior of the cell, we feel that it is important to summarize all further evidence for this concept. Indirect evidence is the two-stage nature of transferrin uptake, the slow rate of transferrin uptake during the second stage and the relatively long mean residence time (about 10 min) of transferrin on the reticulocyte (*Baker* and *Morgan*, 1969b). Other indirect evidence is the observation that sulfhydryl and microtubule reacting agents block not only transferrin uptake but also its release (*Morgan* and *Baker*, 1969; *Hemmaplardh et al.*, 1974) and that ^{59}Fe is not taken up by reticulocytes from transferrin coupled to agarose, latex beads or Enzacryl AA (*Morgan E. H.* – personal communication). Moreover, the observation is important that Fe^{3+} chelating agents have little effect on iron uptake, whereas Fe^{2+} chelating agents which can enter red cells inhibit iron uptake (*Clark* and *Walsh*, 1960; *Morgan*, 1971; *Poňka* and *Neuwirt*, 1970). Finally direct evidence that transferrin does enter the reticulocyte cytoplasm was produced by several authors (*Martinez-Medellin*, 1972; *Martinez-Medellin* and *Schulman*, 1972; *Borová et al.*, 1973; *Sly et al.*, 1975a 1975b; *Neuwirt et al.*, 1975a) who detected labelled transferrin in stroma- and mitochondria-free haemolysate after incubation of reticulocytes with this protein (*see also Sullivan et al.*, 1976).

Despite this evidence some workers doubt the penetration of transferrin into the interior of reticulocytes (*Fielding* and *Speyer*, 1974; *Workman* and *Bates*, 1975). It is, however, of interest that even those refuting the idea of transferrin penetration into the cell (*Speyer* and *Fielding*, 1974; *Fielding* and *Speyer*, 1974) found free transferrin in the membrane-free cytosol of human reticulocytes incubated with transferrin-[125]I. In their experiments the amount of transferrin in cytosol was very small; this, however, does not rule out that the complex of iron with transferrin does not penetrate through the membrane. The relatively small amount of transferrin-^{125}I inside the reticulocyte may be due to the rapid exchange of transferrin molecules.

After giving up its iron, transferrin is released from erythroid cells. If transferrin enters reticulocytes by endocytosis, it seems probable that a transferrin release occurs by a similar process, i.e. exocytosis (*Morgan E. H.*, personal communication).

The exchange of iron between transferrin and erythroid cells of the bone marrow takes place in a manner very similar to that in reticulocytes. The pattern of transferrin and iron uptake by bone marrow cells occurs in four stages: (1) adsorption of transferrin, (2) progressive uptake of transferrin, (3) release of iron to the cell, (4) release of transferrin from the cell. There are, however, quantitative differences, since total transferrin uptake per bone-marrow erythroid-precursor cell is eight times that per reticulocyte and the rate of iron uptake is about twice as great in marrow cells (*Kailis* and *Morgan*, 1974).

FACTORS INFLUENCING IRON UPTAKE BY ERYTHROID CELLS

Iron is taken up by immature red cells in all stages of their development. Autoradiographic studies revealed that the youngest cells take up iron most actively (*Lajtha* and *Suit*, 1955). The capacity to assimilate iron declines gradually with maturation (*Alpen* and *Cranmore*, 1959; *Erslev* and *Hughes*, 1960; *Myhre*, 1964a; *Najean et al.*, 1964) and the transformation of reticulocytes into erythrocytes is associated with a loss of the ability to incorporate iron (*Belcher* and *Courtenay*, 1959). The nature of these changes has not so far been elucidated and it is not yet known whether they are related to the cessation of haemoglobin synthesis. Kinetic studies support the idea that as the erythroid cell matures, the receptor sites for transferrin binding are lost (*Kornfeld*, 1968).

The iron uptake by erythroid precursors of a given maturity depends on two basic factors. The first is the amount of transferrin – iron complex and perhaps also the iron distribution on the transferrin molecule. The second factor is the metabolic state of the cell. The latter depends in particular on the metabolic activity of mitochondria, the membrane structure, which depends on SH groups and functioning microtubule-like proteins, and finally on the relationship between haem and globin synthesis.

Iron and transferrin levels and transferrin saturation

The amount of transferrin bound to reticulocytes rises with increasing concentrations of this protein in the environment. Two distinct phases of this process can be differentiated. At lower physiological transferrin levels the transferrin uptake is specific and reaches its maximum at about 0.05 mM transferrin concentration. The second slower stage of transferrin uptake occurs at transferrin concentrations from 0.1 mM to 0.7 mM. At these higher levels transferrin is bound to cells by non-specific adsorptive processes (*Baker* and *Morgan*, 1969a, 1971).

There are conflicting reports concerning the effect of the degree of transferrin saturation both on transferrin binding to reticulocytes, and on the extent of iron incorporation into reticulocytes. *Jandl* and *Katz* (1963) concluded that human Fe^{3+}-transferrin has a much greater affinity for "receptor" sites on the membrane of human reticulocytes than iron-free transferrin. *Kornfeld's* study (1969) pertaining to the interaction of human transferrin with rabbit reticulocytes supported the view that the binding of metals to apotransferrin affects the binding of the protein with its "receptor" sites. However, transferrin completely saturated with iron had only a slightly higher affinity to reticulocytes than mono-Fe^{3+}-transferrin. On the other hand, *Baker* and *Morgan* (1969b) provided evidence that there is only a very small difference in the affinity of rabbit reticulocytes for iron-saturated or iron-free rabbit transferrin. The same authors assume that iron-containing transferrin molecules have a larger mean residence time on the reticulocyte. The different results are obviously due to different properties of human and rabbit transferrin (*Lane*, 1971, 1972).

20

The binding of iron to human transferrin markedly alters the surface properties of the molecule, while practically no changes are found with rabbit transferrin.

Another problem is the effect of the degree of iron saturation of transferrin on iron uptake by immature erythroid cells. It has been suggested that the iron uptake by reticulocytes depends on the absolute concentration of the iron – transferrin complex, regardless of the relative transferrin saturation (*Schade*, 1961; *Morgan* and *Laurell*, 1963; *Katz* and *Jandl*, 1964). In lower concentrations, the greater the concentration of the complex of iron and transferrin in the environment, the more iron is incorporated into the reticulocytes. At relatively high concentrations a further increase in the iron-transferrin concentration does not influence the iron uptake by reticulocytes. In bone-marrow cells transferrin saturation has, however, a marked effect on iron uptake. *Kailis* and *Morgan* (1974) demonstrated that at a constant iron concentration iron uptake by bone-marrow cells decreased as the transferrin concentration was raised (i.e. saturation decreased).

Fletcher and *Huehns* (1967, 1968) presented a hypothesis that erythroid cells obtain iron preferentially from one binding site of transferrin. *In vitro* studies using rabbit reticulocytes and human transferrin confirmed the observation of *Fletcher* and *Huehns* (*Chernelch* and *Brown*, 1970; *Zapolski et al.*, 1974; *Harris* and *Aisen*, 1975) and supported the view that the two iron binding sites of transferrin are not physiologically equivalent. However, *Williams* and *Woodworth* (1973) working with chick-embryo red cells and conalbumin, and *Harris* and *Aisen* (1975), using rabbit reticulocytes and rabbit transferrin, did not find evidence of a functional difference between the two binding sites of transferrin. As far as experiments *in vivo* are concerned, some attempts to demonstrate differences between the two iron-binding sites were unsuccessful (*Chernelch* and *Brown*, 1970; *Lane* and *Finch*, 1970), while others were successful (*Ganzoni et al.*, 1972; *Hahn*, 1973; *Brown*, 1975). The problem of the functional difference of the two binding sites of transferrin requires further study. Here it is pertinent to point out the view of *Harris* and *Aisen* (1975), that if the functional heterogeneity of specific sites of transferrin has any regulatory function, it should be present in all species. The above mentioned inter-species differences therefore rather interfere with the concept that the functional heterogeneity of two binding sites of transferrin can play a general role in the control of iron transport to erythroid cells.

Metabolic state of erythroid cells

Earlier reports were conflicting with respect to the effect of metabolic inhibitors on iron uptake (*Clark* and *Walsh*, 1959; *Katz* and *Jandl*, 1964). *Morgan* and *Baker* (1969), who contributed considerably to the elucidation of the relationship between energy metabolism and iron uptake, studied the effect of clearly defined metabolic inhibitors. These authors found that all inhibitors of the oxidative metabolism tested (rotenone, 2,4-dinitrophenol, oligomycin, NaCN and NaN$_3$) reduced the iron uptake by reticulocytes more than the uptake of transferrin. Morgan (1971) demonstrated subsequently that these substances inhibit iron release from transferrin in reticulo-cytes. Rotenone and oligomycin inhibit in particular NADH-linked electron transfer and it may be therefore assumed that the flow of electrons from NADH to cytochrome b — which takes place in mitochondria — is essential for the release of iron from trans-ferrin. NADH obviously reduces trivalent iron and at the same time provides a proton for transferrin. In their original work *Morgan* and *Baker* collected indirect evidence against the concept that iron uptake depends simply on high-energy compounds such as ATP. Recently, however, *Morgan* (personal communication) found a very good correlation between the decrease of ATP and the decrease of transferrin and iron uptake. At present this author assumes that it is the ATP concentration which is critical for iron uptake.

The problem of iron release from transferrin in the cell is very complex because cell-free preparations of reticulocytes even in the presence of ATP, ascorbic acid, NADH, citrate and glutathione release iron from transferrin much less readily than intact reticulocytes (*Morgan*, 1971). An integral structure of the erythroid cell seems to be essential for the release of iron from transferrin. The structural integrity of the reticulocyte is also essential for the specific interaction between transferrin and reti-culocytes (*Morgan* and *Baker*, 1974) and it is possible that this interaction must precede the physiological dissociation of the iron—transferrin complex.

Another mechanism seems to be involved during the process of iron release from transferrin by reticulocytes in addition to iron reduction and the provision of a proton to transferrin. It has been suggested that during the biological removal of iron from transferrin an enzymatic attack on the transferrin-bound bicarbonate is essential (*Martinez-Medellin*, 1972; *Egyed*, 1973; *Aisen* and *Leibman*, 1973; *Martinez-Medellin* and *Schulman*, 1973; *Schulman et al.*, 1974). The hypothesis has been presented that protein kinase activated by cyclic AMP is required for the activation of this enzyme (*Poňka* and *Neuwirt*, 1975a). This idea is supported by the observation that the in-hibition of adenylate cyclase or stimulation of phosphodiesterase in reticulocytes is associated with reduction of iron uptake.

The role of sulfhydryl groups in iron uptake

Intact sulfhydryl groups are essential for normal iron uptake by reticulocytes (*Fielding et al.*, 1969; *Morgan* and *Baker*, 1969; *Edwards* and *Fielding*, 1971) because various SH-inhibitors markedly reduce the iron uptake by reticulocytes. *Morgan* and *Baker* (1969) concluded that inhibition of iron uptake after sulfhydryl inhibitors is secondary as a result of primary reduction of transferrin passage into reticulocytes. Sulfhydryl reagents do not influence the transferrin binding to the receptors but almost completely block the phase of progressive transferrin uptake (*van Bocksmeer et al.*, 1975). These inhibitors also reduce the transferrin release from reticulocytes. *Edwards* and *Fielding* (1971) suggested that sulfhydryl groups participate directly in some way in the dissociation of iron from transferrin or are required for the transport of iron from the iron—transferrin—receptor complex (*Fielding* and *Speyer*, 1974). Further experiments are needed to elucidate the conflicting reports of the two groups of authors.

Other factors which influence iron uptake

Wise and *Archdeacon* (1965, 1967) originally suggested that the $Na^+ - K^+$ ATPase system, which can be inhibited by ouabain, participates in the transfer of iron to reticulocytes. On the other hand, *Morgan* and *Baker* (1969) obtained no evidence that ouabain-sensitive membrane ATPase is involved in iron uptake. *Wise* and *Archdeacon* (1969) concluded in their subsequent study that the $Na^+ - K^+$ ATPase system has only a minor effect on the total iron transport. It is, however, possible that it could participate in the movement of iron from the cell membrane into the cell interior.

In recent years numerous substances were described which inhibit the transport of ^{59}Fe into reticulocytes, e.g. ethacrynic acid (*Barnett* and *Archdeacon*, 1970), cycloheximide, emetine, puromycin, fluoride, chloramphenicol, tryptamine, haemin, propranolol, imidazole and other compounds (*Morgan* and *Baker*, 1969; *Poňka* and *Neuwirt*, 1969, 1971, 1975a; *Egyed*, 1974). The mechanism of action of some of these substances has not so far been elucidated. The mechanism of action of haem and protein synthesis inhibitors (cycloheximide, puromycin and emetine) on iron uptake by reticulocytes is of considerable interest and will be discussed later (*see* p. 45).

Iron uptake from chelating agents

The great importance of transferrin results from its ability to prevent indiscriminate iron uptake by various cells and to supply iron to cells synthesizing haemoglobin. The chemical nature of this process has not yet been elucidated. Studies of iron incorporation from synthetic chelating agents represent an interesting approach which can promote the understanding of specific iron uptake for haemoglobin synthesis. On the other hand, investigations of the influence of different chelating agents on iron uptake from transferrin and on haemoglobin synthesis are important for elucidating the intracellular kinetics of iron.

Cleton, Turnbull and *Finch* (1963) provided evidence that radioiron bound to ethylenediaminedi-(*o*-hydroxyphenyl)-acetic acid (EDHA) was delivered to reticulocytes and that 50–90% of the ^{59}Fe taken up was incorporated into haemoglobin. *Princiotto et al.* (1964) and *Morgan* (1971) confirmed that reticulocytes can utilize iron bound to several low-molecular-weight iron-complexing agents (chelating agents). In the majority of instances reticulocytes utilized more readily iron bound to transferrin than iron bound to chelating agents for haemoglobin synthesis. However, certain chelating agents [citrate, nitrilotriacetic acid, N-β-hydroxyethylimino-diacetic acid (HEDA)] supplied iron practically as readily as transferrin. Certain

23

features are common to uptake of iron bound to chelating agents and iron associated with transferrin. Both processes are highly temperature-dependent and can be blocked by inhibitors of oxidative metabolism (*Morgan*, 1971). Moreover, the rate at which iron is supplied from chelating agents to reticulocytes is directly related to the rate at which iron is exchanged between chelating agents and transferrin. It seems thus obvious that the mechanism of iron uptake by reticulocytes from the synthetic iron chelating agents is dependent on an initial exchange of iron from the chelating agents to transferrin present in the cells. This idea was confirmed by elegant experiments of *Hemmaplardh* and *Morgan* (1974) who demonstrated that the removal of transferrin from reticulocytes considerably reduces the ability of cells to take up iron from chelating agents.

INTRACELLULAR KINETICS OF IRON

In vitro studies suggest the presence of non-haem intermediates on the pathway of iron to the haemoglobin molecule inside the immature erythroid cell. The main problem when tracing the intracellular fate of iron ensues from the fact that non-haem iron inside the erythroid cells, whether estimated chemically or with the use of isotopes, need not represent the necessary intermediary pool between transferrin and haem.

There is direct and indirect evidence of non-haem iron in immature erythroid cells. It is known that the youngest recognizable erythroblasts take up Fe (*Lajtha* and *Suit*, 1955) although these erythroid elements contain only negligible amounts of haemoglobin (*Thorell*, 1962; *Borsook*, 1964). *In vitro* studies with reticulocytes indicate that radioiron passes through a minor non-haem iron pool which is located between plasma transferrin and haem. *Nejean et al.* (1967) observed that radioiron enters reticulocytes in a linear fashion, while its incorporation into haem is somewhat delayed. The relationship between the incorporation of radioiron into reticulocytes and haem can be expressed quantitatively by a relatively simple method. It is possible to calculate the percentage of total iron incorporated into reticulocytes which appears in haem during incubation *in vitro* (*Poňka* and *Neuwirt*, 1969). In this way the distribution of radioiron in haem and non-haem pool of reticulocytes can be investigated at different time intervals (*see* Fig. 9, p. 37). After a certain time an equilibrium is established between the haem and non-haem pool of radioiron and even in the course of further incubation $40-20\%$ ^{59}Fe taken up by the cell remain in the non-haem pool. A similar approach was independently used by *Ganzoni* in 1968. The relatively high percentage of non-haem radioiron observed in reticulocytes incubated *in vitro* is most probably due to unphysiological conditions occurring in experiments *in vitro* (*Myhre*, 1964b).

Direct evidence of the presence of non-haem iron in immature erythroid cells was provided by electronmicroscopic (*Bessis*, 1963), microspectrophotometric (*Sondhaus* and *Thorell*, 1960) and electrophoretic (*Falbe-Hansen* and *Lothe*, 1962) studies. The detailed work of *Allen* and *Jandl* (1960) concerned with the intracellular kinetics of iron in rabbit reticulocytes showed the presence of a non-haemoglobin protein which binds ^{59}Fe.

After 1960 attention was mainly focused on investigations of the chemical nature of different non-haem proteins and iron complexes.

Ferritin

Ferritin, discovered by *Laufberger* (1936, 1937), is the main form in which iron is stored in the reticuloendothelial system. The large molecule has a diameter of 100 to 110 Å and a molecular weight of cca 400,000–500,000 daltons. Inside the protein shell are trivalent iron micelles which may account for as much as 23% of the weight of ferritin. By reduction of Fe^{3+} with cystein, glutathione, or ascorbic acid, iron (II) is released and the protein component apoferritin remains, the latter being made up of 20 identical polypeptide chains (*Harrison*, 1964). Under the electron microscope ferritin can also be detected in erythroblasts; its amount declines, however, with advancing maturity of the erythroid cell and it is not present in circulating red cells (*Bessis*, 1963). Ferritin molecules are present mainly in the cytoplasm. In some hypochromic hypersideraemic anaemias there is an excessive amount of ferritin in immature erythroid cells (*Bessis* and *Breton-Gorius*, 1959; *Bessis*, 1963; *Bessis* and *Jensen*, 1965; *Goodman* and *Hall*, 1967; *see also* p. 168) or in reticular cells (*Tanaka*, 1967). It is worth mentioning that ferritin is not found in avian erythroblasts (*F. R. Campbell* quoted by *Krantz* and *Jacobson*, 1970).

Morphological research elucidated neither the origin of ferritin in erythroblasts nor the problem of the possible utilization of ferritin iron for haem synthesis. Several later studies proved unequivocally that direct synthesis can be the main source of ferritin in erythroid cells (*Mazur* and *Carleton*, 1963; *Zail et al.*, 1964; *Matioli* and *Eylar*, 1964). *De novo* synthesis of apoferritin* is found only in erythroid cells of the bone marrow and disappears during maturation of reticulocytes. Erythroid cells at all stages of maturation including reticulocytes are, however, able to incorporate iron into ferritin (*Yamada* and *Gabudza*, 1974a).

Electrophoretic research of ferritin in bone-marrow elements differentiated two components with a different mobility. Bone-marrow ferritin having a greater mobility originates in erythroblasts, while slow marrow ferritin comes from reticuloendothelial cells (*Alfrey et al.*, 1967; *Gabudza* and *Gardner*, 1967). Rapidly migrating erythroblast ferritin of the bone marrow obtains iron mainly from transferrin, while ferritin iron which migrates more slowly comes from broken down erythrocytes. The first type was therefore denoted as "anabolic" and the second as "catabolic" ferritin (*Gabudza* and *Pearson*, 1968, 1969).

*i.e. apoferritin specific for erythroblasts

As far as the role of ferritin iron in haemoglobin synthesis is concerned, *Mazur* and *Carleton* (1963) and *Fielding* and *Speyer* (1975) assume that ferritin is an essential intermediate for iron transfer to the haem molecule. This view was, however, not generally accepted and the majority of authors assume that ferritin takes up iron only if more iron enters the cell than is required by the actual rate of haem synthesis (*Zail et al.*, 1964; *Primosigh* and *Thomas*, 1968; *Borová et al.*, 1973; *see also* p. 33). Since ferritin iron does not serve as a substrate for haem synthesis (*Yoneyama et al.*, 1963; *Malinowska et al.*, 1964), it was suggested that this protein leaves reticulocytes before they mature (*Zail et al.*, 1964). *Deiss* and *Cartwright* (1970) actually demonstrated in experiments with swine reticulocytes the movement of ferritin from erythroid cells into plasma and from there into monocytes. This process requires functional mitochondria and is relatively rapid (within hours). Plasma contains natural antibodies against ferritin from erythroblasts which perhaps play a part in the ferritin transfer between erythroid precursor cells and RE cells (*Yamada* and *Gabudza*, 1974b).

There certainly exists a relationship between the rate of haemoglobin synthesis and the ferritin content of immature erythroid cells. An increased amount of ferritin was demonstrated in hypochromic hypersideraemic anaemias (*Bessis* and *Breton-Gorius*, 1959; *Bessis* and *Jensen*, 1965), where the rate of haem synthesis is reduced (*see* p. 168). In erythroid cells with inhibited haemoglobin synthesis enhanced ferritin synthesis was described (*Eylar* and *Matioli*, 1965; *Matioli* and *Eylar*, 1964).

Other non-haem iron proteins and iron complexes

In addition to ferritin immature erythroid cells contain other non-haemoglobin proteins which were isolated by electrophoresis or chromatography (*Allen* and *Jandl*, 1960; *Salera et al.*, 1961; *Greenough et al.*, 1962; *Zail et al.*, 1964; *Primosigh* and *Thomas*, 1968; *Borová et al.*, 1973; *Speyer* and *Fielding*, 1974; *Fielding* and *Speyer*, 1974; *Workman* and *Bates*, 1974, 1975). *Greenough, Zail, Primosigh* and their collaborators found during incubation of immature erythroid cells early incorporation of ^{59}Fe into the haemolysate fraction which was eluated from an amberlite resin as the first peak and was described as fraction I. *Greenough et al.* (1962) concluded that fraction I resembles globin. When it binds iron, so-called "sideroglobin" is formed which is the common precursor of both protein and iron component of the haemoglobin molecule. This idea has never been confirmed.

Speyer and *Fielding* (1974) subjected the water soluble (cytosol) fraction of human reticulocytes to chromatography on Sephadex G-200 and differentiated haemoglobin and component C, which they identified later as ferritin. In the stroma dissolved in Triton X-100, separated on Sepharose 2B and 6B, they found three iron-bearing components which they described as A, B$_1$ and B$_2$. Component B$_2$ has a molecular weight of 230,000 daltons and seems to be a complex of iron and transferrin bound with the receptor. The membrane component A has not been characterized in more detail. It is, however, surprising that more iron ^{59}Fe was incorporated into component

26

A than into haemoglobin. These authors consider component B_1 speculatively as the membrane iron-transport intermediate (*Fielding* and *Speyer*, 1974).

Workman and *Bates* (1974, 1975) identified recently in the cytosol of reticulocytes a protein with a molecular weight of 5,000 daltons which in their opinion serves for iron transport from the transferrin receptor site on the membrane into the haem molecule. This component, described as "siderochelin", can also give up its iron to ferritin in the cytosol. ATP enhances iron transport from the membrane in the presence of stroma-free cytosol, but is not part of "siderochelin". However, evidence against the possible role of "siderochelin" in intracellular iron transport can be taken from the following experiment. ^{59}Fe-labelled "siderochelin" incubated with fresh mitochondria-free reticulocyte lysate can give up all its iron to haemoglobin. This finding cannot be explained satisfactorily, since haem synthetase — which is present in mitochondria — is essential for iron incorporation into haem (*see* p. 66). Recently *Blackburn* and *Morgan* (in press), using the same experimental approach have concluded that the low molecular weight iron-binding component of the cytosol of reticulocytes is not essential for the release of iron from the reticulocyte stroma.

Another point, which is not clear, is whether there exists a low-molecular intermediate of iron in the cytosol. *Martinez-Medellin* and *Schulman* (1972) used ultrafiltration (on Amicon UM-10 membrane) and obtained no evidence for the existence of iron in a low-molecular form. Other authors using chromatographic techniques or polyacrylamide gel electrophoresis demonstrated, however, low-molecular iron in bone-marrow cells (*Primosigh* and *Thomas*, 1968; *Storring* and *Fatih*, 1975) or in reticulocytes (*Borová et al.*, 1973). So far no agreement has been reached whether or not low-molecular-weight iron is a metabolic intermediate in the iron transport into the haem molecule (*Borová et al.*, 1973; *Storring* and *Fatih*, 1975).

Mitochondrial iron

Mitochondria, where iron is incorporated into haem, are the final destination of iron in the erythroid cell (*Sano et al.*, 1959; *Cooper et al.*, 1963; *London et al.*, 1964; *Harris*, 1964). The form in which iron enters mitochondria and in which it is present in mitochondria is not known. It is possible that iron is bound to ATP and other nucleotides (*Mazur et al.*, 1960; *Goucher* and *Taylor*. 1964; *Konopka et al.*, 1969; *Konopka* and *Szotor*, 1972), sucrose (*Romslo*, 1974) or other intracellular chelating agents. The iron uptake by mitochondria *in vitro* depends on time and temperature (*Cooper et al.*, 1963) and takes place by two different mechanism, i.e. by an energy-independent and energy-dependent mechanism (*Romslo*, 1974). Copper or an enzyme dependent on this metal is essential for iron transport into mitochondria of immature red cells (*Goodman* and *Dallman*, 1960; *Williams et al.*, 1976). Sonicated mitochondria are able to catalyze the reduction of ferric salts and subsequently to incorporate ferrous iron into haem. The ability to reduce iron is a property of the inner mitochondrial membrane, probably in proximity of haem synthetase. Possible sites of this reduction are flavoproteins, succinate and NADH dehydrogenase (*Barnes et al.*, 1972). The results with isolated mitochondria must, however, be evaluated with great caution as the integrity of the cell is lost. Cell integrity is essential for normal intracellular iron metabolism (*Morgan*, 1971; *Morgan* and *Baker*, 1974). Moreover, in work with artificial cell-free systems mitochondria are not necessarily supplied with a natural source of iron.

Inhibitors of haem synthesis as a tool in investigations of the intracellular kinetics of iron

Understanding of the kinetics of iron from extracellular transferrin into the haemoglobin molecule is facilitated by various inhibitors of this transport. The effect of some of them e.g. of inhibitors of sulfhydryl groups has not been completely elucidated (*see* p. 22). There exist, however, inhibitors of haem synthesis which have a known mechanism of action and which proved useful in investigations of the intracellular

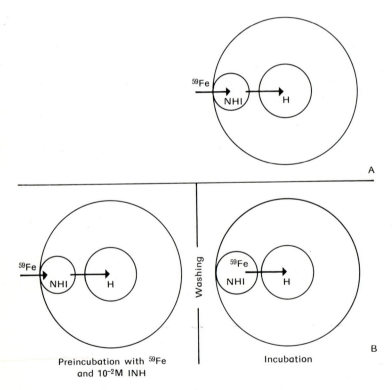

Fig. 2. Scheme of incorporation of radioiron into haem from transferrin and from intracellular non-haem iron pool (NHI — non-haem pool of iron; H — haem pool of iron). (A) Synthesis of haem from transferrin-bound ^{59}Fe; (B) synthesis of haem from non-haem ^{59}Fe. (From *Poňka* and *Neuwirt*, 1970. Reproduced with the permission of Blackwell Scientific Publications Ltd., Oxford.)

iron metabolism as well as in investigations of the regulation of haem synthesis in integrated reticulocytes.

It has been long well established that lead inhibits haem synthesis; since it does not reduce cellular iron uptake, lead induces the accumulation of iron in non-haem forms (*Jandl et al.*, 1959; *Zail et al.*, 1964; *Primosigh* and *Thomas*, 1968; *Poňka* and *Neuwirt*, 1969). Another obviously more specific inhibitor of haem synthesis is isonicotinic acid hydrazide (INH). INH is an antagonist of pyridoxine (*Biehl* and *Vilter*, 1954) which is a co-factor of δ-aminolaevulinic acid synthetase (*see* p. 59). Addition of INH to reticulocytes incubated *in vitro* inhibits haem synthesis assessed by ^{59}Fe and glycine-2-^{14}C incorporation; radioactivity of ^{59}Fe in whole cells, however, does not change or even increases (*Poňka* and *Neuwirt*, 1969, 1971; *see* Fig. 10, 14).

Fig. 2 illustrates the design of the experiment which was used to resolve the question whether non-haem iron-^{59}Fe present in reticulocytes after preincubation with

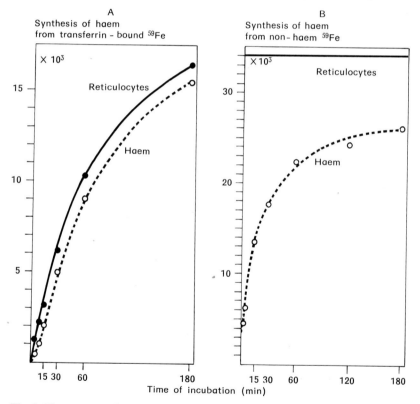

Fig. 3. Time course of radioactivity in reticulocytes with radio-iron bound: A, to plasma transferrin; B, in intracellular non-haem pool of reticulocytes. Ordinates: cpm of ^{59}Fe incorporated per 0.2 ml of reticulocytes — solid line; cpm of ^{59}Fe incorporated into the total haem present in 0.2 ml of reticulocytes — broken line. (From *Poňka* and *Neuwirt*, 1970. Reproduced with the permission of Blackwell Scientific Publications Ltd., Oxford.)

transferrin-^{59}Fe and INH can be utilized for haem synthesis during subsequent incubation. Fig. 3A shows the incorporation of transferrin-bound radioiron into reticulocytes and haem. The radioactivity of ^{59}Fe increases during incubation in reticulocytes as well as in haem. Fig. 3B demonstrates the ^{59}Fe-radioactivity in haem and reticulocytes which had previously been preincubated with 10^{-2}M INH and transferrin-^{59}Fe. The radioactivity of reticulocytes does not change in the course of the second incubation. On the other hand, the radioactivity of haem increases during the subsequent three-hour incubation. Details pertaining to the experimental technique have been described elsewhere (*Poňka* and *Neuwirt*, 1970).

The importance of preincubation in the presence of INH is shown clearly by the following experiment (Fig. 4). Two groups of reticulocytes were preincubated with

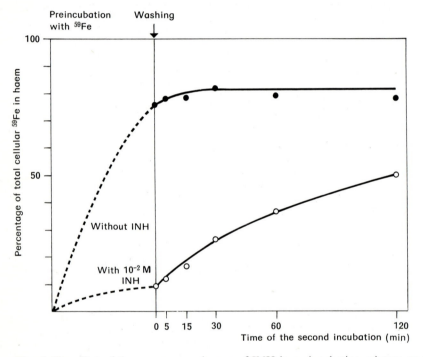

Fig. 4. The effect of the presence or absence of INH in preincubation mixture on the cellular distribution of radioiron in the course of the second incubation. (From *Poňka* and *Neuwirt*, 1970. Reproduced with the permission of Blackwell Scientific Publications Ltd. Oxford.)

plasma containing ^{59}Fe and to one group INH was added. After thorough rinsing the cells were reincubated. In reticulocytes preincubated without INH the percentage of radioiron in haem was much greater immediately after the first incubation. During the second incubation the radioactivity of haem in this group of reticulocytes showed

30

practically no further increase. Fig. 4 clearly shows that in reticulocytes preincubated with INH there is much more intracellular non-haem radioiron available for haem synthesis during the second incubation.

For the correct interpretation of these chase experiments it is essential to know whether preincubation with INH impairs the capacity of reticulocytes to form haem and whether preincubated reticulocytes have an altered ability to take up radioiron from transferrin. From Fig. 5 it follows that reticulocytes with a high non-radioactive iron content in the non-haem pool (after preincubation with INH and cold iron)

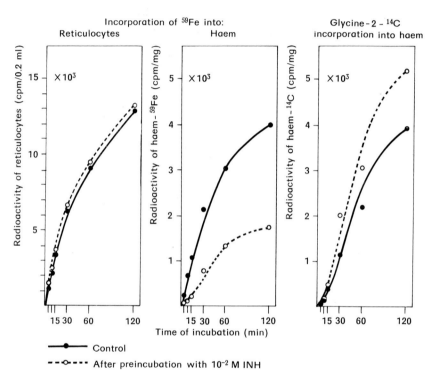

Fig. 5. The uptake of iron and its incorporation into haem of reticulocytes preincubated for 60 minutes with or without 10^{-2} M INH and with plasma-bound ^{56}Fe and the incorporation of glycine-2-^{14}C into haem of both types of cells. Medium used for the second incubation contained 1/4 of rabbit plasma. (From *Poňka* and *Neuwirt*, 1970. Reproduced with the permission of Blackwell Scientific Publications Ltd., Oxford.)

do not have a reduced ability to take up radioiron from transferrin. Incorporation of ^{59}Fe into the haem of preincubated reticulocytes is much lower than in normal cells (*see* Fig. 5). Radioiron which enters cells preincubated with INH is diluted (i.e. its specific activity declines) in the large pool of non-radioactive non-haem iron. Conversely the presence of non-radioactive plasma iron in the incubation mixture during the second incubation (without INH and ^{59}Fe) reduces the utilization of radioiron from the non-haem pool. This finding can be explained by a drop of the specific activity of intracellular non-haem radioiron which resulted from dilution with non-labelled iron from plasma transferrin (*Poňka* and *Neuwirt*, 1970).

Haem synthesis in reticulocytes preincubated with INH is, however, not impaired, perhaps it is even enhanced, as apparent from the higher incorporation of glycine-2-^{14}C into the haem of reticulocytes preincubated with INH (*see* Fig. 5, last curve on the right).

The results with specific inhibitors of haem synthesis which inhibit the transfer of radioiron from the non-haem pool to haem (Table 1) provide evidence that incorporation of radioiron into haem is due to haem synthesis during the second

Table 1

Effect of various inhibitors on the utilization of transferrin-bound and intracellular non-haem radioiron for haem synthesis; each value represents the mean value of four samples $\pm$ S.D.

| | Incorporation of ^{59}Fe into haem from: | | | |
| | Reticulocyte non-haem iron pool | | Transferrin | |
	cpm $\pm$ S.D.	%	cpm $\pm$ S.D.	%
Control	4,318 $\pm$ 133	100.0	3,815 $\pm$ 359	100.0
10^{-3}M INH	2,698 $\pm$ 36	62.5	3,674 $\pm$ 236	96.3
Control	1,747 $\pm$ 220	100.0	4,762 $\pm$ 209	100.0
10^{-3}M bipyridyl	699 $\pm$ 160	40.0	31 $\pm$ 29	0.7

(From *Poňka* and *Neuwirt*, 1970. Reproduced with the permission of Blackwell Scientific Publications Ltd., Oxford.)

incubation. This method is important in particular because it enables us to differentiate primary inhibition of haem synthesis from primary inhibition of iron uptake by the reticulocyte. It is obvious that if some substance interferes with the iron uptake by reticulocytes and does not directly inhibit haem synthesis, the specific activity of haem does not change in an experimental set-up where intracellular non-haem iron-^{59}Fe is utilized for haem synthesis (*see* Fig. 2). Another advantage of this method is that it makes possible the evaluation of the influence of various factors on haem synthesis in the intact erythroid cell (*see* p. 82).

The above experimental approach can also contribute to deeper understanding of the complicated kinetics of iron in immature red cell precursors (*Borová et al.*,

1973; *Storring* and *Fatih*, 1975; *Fielding* and *Speyer*, 1975; *Neuwirt et al.*, 1975a). Incubation of reticulocytes with INH increases the radioactivity of ^{59}Fe most significantly in the stroma* and also in the low-molecular fraction and non-haemoglobin proteins (Fig. 6) (*Borová et al.*, 1973). However, INH does neither increase the amount

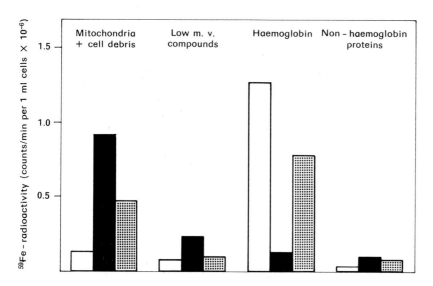

Fig. 6. Distribution of ^{59}Fe-radioactivity in rabbit reticulocytes after 1 h of incubation with ^{59}Fe bound to rabbit plasma transferrin. Reticulocytes were incubated under standard incubation conditions and further treated, as described in *Borová et al.* (1973). The chase experiment in which intracellular non-haem iron is re-utilized for haem synthesis was performed, as described in *Poňka* and *Neuwirt* (1970). Empty columns, control reticulocytes; black columns, reticulocytes incubated with INH; dotted columns, reticulocytes re-incubated after removal of INH. For details see *Borová et al.* (1973). (Reproduced with the permission of Elsevier/North-Holland Biomedical Press B.V., Amsterdam.)

of transferrin in the stroma fraction nor in the cytosol. Further analysis revealed that practically all ^{59}Fe accumulated in the "stroma" after INH treatment is mitochondrial radioiron (*Borová et al.*, 1973). The increase of radioactivity in non-haemoglobin proteins of reticulocytes incubated with INH is due to the great ^{59}Fe accumulation in ferritin. During reincubation of reticulocytes after removal of INH and labelled iron no decrease of the specific activity of ^{59}Fe ferritin was observed. In such a chase experiment, however, the amount of radioiron in haemoglobin rises (*Poňka* and *Neuwirt*, 1970) (Fig. 3B and 4) at the expense of ^{59}Fe in the low-molecular fraction and mitochondria (*Borová et al.*, 1973). The above experiments show that during

*This fraction contains mitochondria plus membranes.

33

inhibited haem synthesis iron is readily released from transferrin and a great proportion of the released iron enters the mitochondria. After removal of the inhibitor of haem synthesis the iron accumulated in mitochondria rapidly associates with protoporphyrin IX and is released from the mitochondria as haem (*Borová et al.*, 1973; *Poňka et al.*, 1973b).

Despite the fact that an immense amount of experimental data has been assembled in recent years, it is still not possible to establish the exact pathway of iron from extracellular transferrin into the haem molecule in the immature erythroid cell. It should be pointed out that there are basically two concepts. One is based on experiments by *Morgan* and collaborators (*Morgan* and *Baker*, 1969; *Morgan* and *Appleton*, 1969; *Morgan*, 1974) and also supported by the results of other authors (*Martinez-Medellin* and *Schulman*, 1972; *Borová et al.*, 1973; *Neuwirt et al.*, 1975a). According to this theory transferrin enters the cell by a process of surface endocytosis; probably it is released from endocytic vesicles and enters the cytoplasm. It is not known whether transferrin remains bound to the receptor in the cytoplasm or is released. It is not even known where iron is released and what is its chemical nature after release nor whether iron is released from free transferrin or transferrin bound to a receptor. There is evidence that the complex of iron and transferrin can associate with mitochondria of reticulocytes (*Neuwirt et al.*, 1975a; *Martinez-Medellin*, 1972) and the possibility must be considered that iron is released from transferrin at this organelle. If this is the case, then both the existence of low-molecular-weight iron pool and the incorporation of iron into ferritin in erythroid cells are difficult to explain. There is, however, a possibility that could bridge these discrepancies: transferrin donates its iron directly to mitochondria and iron in the low-molecular-weight compartment, as well as in ferritin and perhaps in other proteins originates from mitochondria (*Poňka et al.* 1977b).

According to the alternative theory, iron is released from transferrin bound to the membrane receptor and by means of a system of different membrane and cytoplasmatic carriers it penetrates into the haem molecule (*Speyer* and *Fielding*, 1974; *Fielding* and *Speyer*, 1974; *Workman* and *Bates*, 1974, 1975).

Finally it must be emphasized that the intracellular kinetics of iron in erythroblasts may differ considerably from that in reticulocytes. This difference is probably particularly important in the most immature erythroid elements which take up iron but form practically no haemoglobin.

REGULATION OF IRON SUPPLY FOR HAEMOGLOBIN SYNTHESIS

The dependence of iron uptake into the erythroid cell on haem or haemoglobin concentration in the cell or on the rate of their synthesis has not been studied in detail till recently. *Katz* (1965, 1970) concluded that the rate of iron uptake is not controlled by the rate of haemoglobin synthesis, as it is possible to inhibit haem formation by means of lead without restricting the cellular iron uptake. On the other hand, it is known that inhibitors of globin synthesis (*Erslev* and *Iossifides*, 1962; *Ward*, 1966; *Felicetti et al.*, 1966) reduce the uptake of iron by immature erythroid cells. This reduced iron uptake was explained either by the direct effect of the inhibitor on the membrane (*Erslev* and *Iossifides*, 1962) or by inhibited haem synthesis (*Felicetti et al.*, 1966). The latter explanation is obviously incompatible with the known effect of lead on iron uptake and haem synthesis.

In our experiments we investigated in detail the effect of haem and globin synthesis inhibitors on iron uptake by reticulocytes. Considerable attention was devoted to the effect of haem which is generally considered the primary inhibitor of haem synthesis at the level of δ-aminoleavulinic acid synthetase (*London et al.*, 1964; *Lascelles*, 1968, p. 74). The results which are analyzed in detail below indicate that the level of non-haemoglobin haem is the limiting factor of iron uptake by the immature erythroid cell. This fact indicates that the actively metabolizing erythroid cell possesses a specific regulatory mechanism which controls iron uptake.

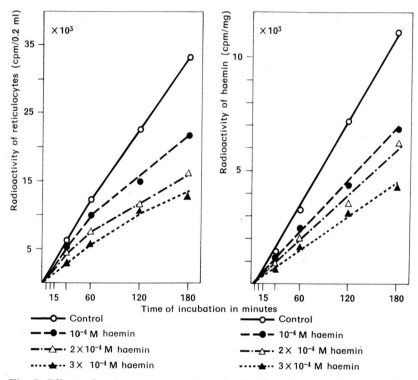

Fig. 7. Effects of various concentrations of added haemin on the incorporation of ^{59}Fe into reticulocytes and on the synthesis of haem. Cells had been preincubated for 20 min with haemin. (From *Poňka* and *Neuwirt* 1969. Reproduced with the permission of Grune and Stratton, Inc., New York.)

Effect of haem on iron uptake by reticulocytes

Addition of haem to intact reticulocytes incubated *in vitro* inhibits not only iron incorporation into haem but also reduces iron uptake by these cells (Fig. 7). Although it was originally reported (*Poňka* and *Neuwirt*, 1969) that haemin exerts its inhibitory effect in concentrations of the order of 10^{-4}M, subsequent results revealed that a concentration of 10^{-5}M is sufficient to reduce the uptake of iron by reticulocytes (Fig. 8). This difference is due to the presence of plasma which was added to the in-

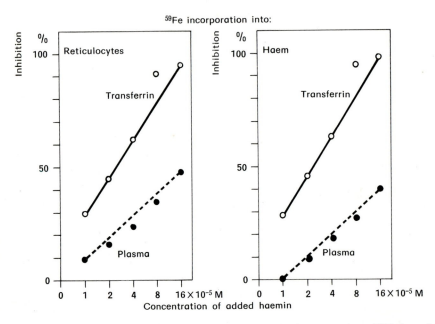

Fig. 8. The effect of various haemin concentrations on the incorporation of ^{59}Fe bound to plasma or purified transferrin into reticulocytes and haem. (From *Poňka* and *Neuwirt*, 1972. Reproduced with the permission of the Birkhäuser Verlag, Basle.)

cubation medium in the first experiments (e.g. in the experiment in Fig. 7). If radio-iron bound to purified transferrin is added to the incubation system, the effective haemin concentration is much lower as the medium does not contain plasma which binds haem (*Poňka* and *Neuwirt*, 1972).

Reduced incorporation of radioiron into reticulocytes incubated with haemin may result from a reduced haem synthesis or may also be due to primary interference of haemin with iron uptake. The former possibility can apply only if the entry of iron into erythroid cells is directly related to the rate of haem synthesis as assumed e.g. by *Gallo* (1967) when interpreting his results. There exists, however, ample evidence

36

that inhibition of haem synthesis is not associated with reduced iron uptake by reticulocytes. First, *in vitro* studies revealed that lead (*see* p. 35), isonicotinic acid hydrazide (Fig. 9) or penicillamine (*see* Fig. 14) inhibit haem synthesis without reducing the uptake of iron by cells. Secondly, in sideroblastic anaemia, where haem synthesis is

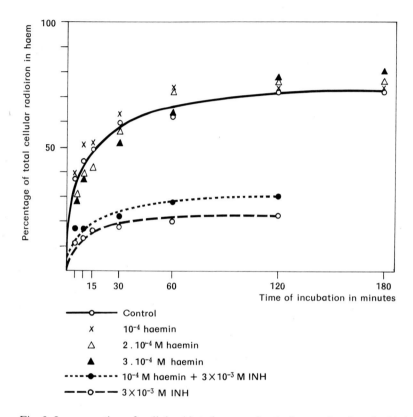

Fig. 9. Incorporation of radioiron into haem and reticulocytes incubated with isonicotinic acid hydrazide and haemin. Cells had been preincubated with INH and haemin for 30 minutes before radioiron was added. (From *Poňka* and *Neuwirt*, 1969. Reproduced with the permission of Grune and Stratton, Inc., New York.)

reduced (*see* p. 168), there is a marked non-haem iron overload in bone-marrow erythroblasts and sometimes in erythrocytes of peripheral blood. These data provide clear evidence that the reduced incorporation of ^{59}Fe into reticulocytes after addition of haemin is not due to reduced haem formation. Haemin obviously interferes with iron uptake by reticulocytes.

In this connection it must be emphasized that exogenous haemin does not reduce the amount of radioiron in haem if the total amount of ^{59}Fe in the reticulocyte is taken into account (Fig. 9). In other words haemin proportionately reduces the radioactivity of ^{59}Fe in reticulocytes and in haem. On the other hand, the specific inhibitor of haem synthesis — INH — inhibits to a considerable extent the utilization of radioiron for haem synthesis by the cell (*see* Fig. 10).

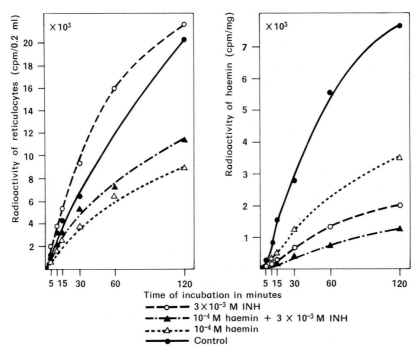

Fig. 10. Time course of cellular distribution of radioiron during *in vitro* incubation of control reticulocytes and of reticulocytes incubated with various inhibitors of haem synthesis. (From *Poňka* and *Neuwirt*, 1969. Reproduced with the permission of Grune and Stratton, Inc., New York.)

Effect of inhibitors of haem and globin syntheses on iron uptake

Experiments where exogenous haemin is added to intact reticulocytes most probably simulate physiological conditions (*Neuwirt et al.*, 1971). Despite this they by no means provide final evidence that intracellular endogenous haem participates in the control of iron uptake. Recent experiments demonstrated the existence of a pool of free haem inside immature erythroid cells (*Neuwirt et al.*, 1972, *see also* p. 136). The amount of intracellular free haem can be considerably increased by incubation with inhibitors of globin synthesis. Conversely inhibitors of haem synthesis prevent the incorporation of labelled substrates into free haem and it may be assumed that they reduce its concentration in the cell.

In subsequent experiments the iron uptake by reticulocytes, incubated with substances which change the size of the endogenous haem pool, was investigated. The results support unequivocally the idea of a regulatory role of haem in iron uptake by reticulocytes.

The kinetics of iron incorporation into reticulocytes as well as into haem after cycloheximide is strikingly similar to the situation which develops during incubation of reticulocytes with haemin (Fig. 11). Similar results were obtained when puromycin

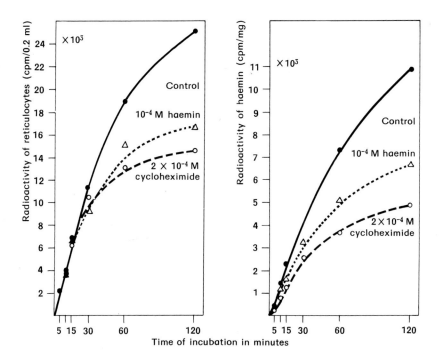

Fig. 11. Comparison of effects of cycloheximide and haemin on the reticulocyte radioiron uptake and on haem synthesis. (From *Poňka* and *Neuwirt*, 1969. Reproduced with the permission of Grune and Stratton, Inc., New York.)

or emetine were used as inhibitors of globin synthesis (*see* below). The effects of cycloheximide and puromycin at the level of ribosomal protein synthesis are very well known (*Beard et al.*, 1969). Emetine inhibits protein synthesis by a similar mechanism as cycloheximide (*Grollman*, 1966, 1968). It seems very probable that free haem,* which accumulates during inhibited globin synthesis, is responsible for the diminished iron uptake into reticulocytes. This idea is strongly supported by the observations that haem synthesis inhibitors (INH and penicillamine) reduce the inhibition of iron uptake by reticulocytes caused by cycloheximide, puromycin or emetine (Fig. 12, 13 and 14). INH, similarly as penicillamine (*du Vigneaud et al.*, 1957), interferes with pyridoxal phosphate which is an essential co-factor in early stages of haem synthesis (p. 59).

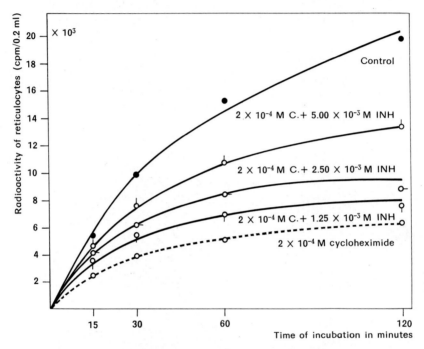

Fig. 12. Incorporation of ^{59}Fe into cycloheximide-treated reticulocytes and into reticulocytes treated with inhibitors of both haem and globin synthesis (INH and cycloheximide). (From *Poňka* and *Neuwirt*, 1969. Reproduced with the permission of Grune and Stratton, Inc. New York.)

*During inhibited globin synthesis the amount of free haem rises as well as of haem bound to non-haemo-globin proteins (*Neuwirt et al.*, 1972), and haem also accumulates in mitochondria (*Poňka, Borová* and *Neuwirt*, 1973b). It is not clear in which form haem exerts its regulatory action. Recently *Koller et al.* (1976) reported that haemin (at concentrations similar to those necessary to depress the release of iron from transferrin by erythroid cells) inhibits the energy-dependent release of iron from transferrin by isolated rat liver mitochondria. It is therefore tempting to speculate that the level of "uncommited" haem (*Israels et al.*, 1975) in mitochondria is the critical factor regulating the rate of iron release from transferrin. Haem in mitochondria might reversibly inhibit the enzymatic system required for the release of iron from transferrin (*see* p. 49)

All the above results are consistent with idea that inhibition of iron uptake by reticulocytes with inhibited protein synthesis depends on the ability of cells to form haem. Experiments with pyridoxal phosphate which restores haem synthesis inhibited by INH (Fig. 15) provide further evidence for this concept. Reticulocytes with inhibited globin synthesis were incubated either with INH alone or with INH and

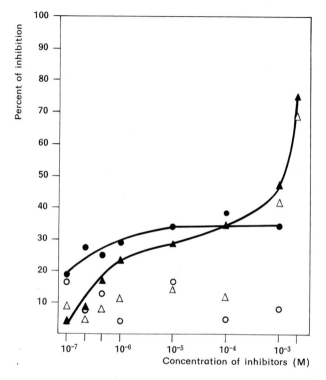

Fig. 13. The effect of INH on the inhibited reticulocyte radioiron uptake caused by various concentrations of cycloheximide or puromycin. Two samples in each group were incubated for 1 h with radioiron after approximately 15-min preincubation with appropriate inhibitors. ●–●. cycloheximide; ○—○, cycloheximide + $5 . 10^{-3}$ M INH; ▲–▲, puromycin; △—△, puromycin + $5 . 10^{-3}$ M INH. (From *Poňka* and *Neuwirt*, 1971. Reproduced with the permission of Elsevier/North-Holland Biomedical Press B.V., Amsterdam.)

pyridoxal phosphate (Fig. 16). The results indicate that the inhibition or restoration of haem synthesis in reticulocytes with inhibited globin synthesis is associated with an increase or decrease of cellular iron uptake respectively.

It appears that iron uptake by reticulocytes does not depend on the actual rate of haemoglobin synthesis but rather on the relationship between haem and globin synthesis. It may be concluded that the rate of iron uptake is inversely proportional to the concentration of free (or uncommitted) haem in the reticulocyte cytoplasm or mitochondria. Such a reversible inhibition by the end-product is a typical feature of feedback systems. The finding of the minor stimulation of iron uptake by reticulocytes incubated with inhibitors of haem synthesis (*see* Fig. 10) can be also explained

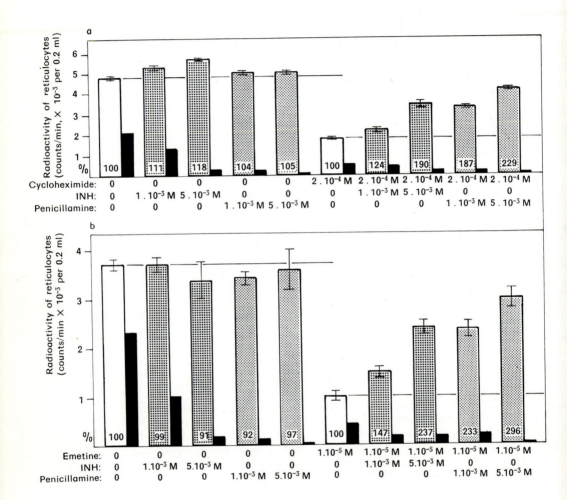

Fig. 14. The effect of various concentrations of INH or penicillamine on the 60-minute uptake of iron by normal reticulocytes or by reticulocytes incubated with cycloheximide (a) or emetine (b). The numbers in columns indicate percentages of appropriate controls. The narrow black columns reveal the incorporation of radioiron into haem (in counts/min per mg) of reticulocytes incubated with or without indicated inhibitors. Each column represents a mean of three (experiment with cycloheximide) or four (experiment with emetine) values $\pm$S.D. (From *Poňka* and *Neuwirt*, 1971. Reproduced with the permission of Elsevier/North-Holland Biomedical Press B.V., Amsterdam.)

42

by a reduction of free (uncommitted) haem which is also present in normal reticulocytes (*Neuwirt et al.*, 1972).

Several authors confirmed recently the inhibitory role of haem in iron uptake by reticulocytes (*Schulman et al.*, 1974; *Fielding* and *Speyer*, 1975). Moreover, *Koller et al.* (1976) demonstrated that haemin reduces the energy-dependent iron uptake by mitochondria in a cell-free system prepared from rat liver. It must be emphasized

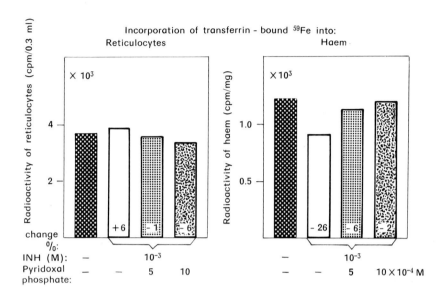

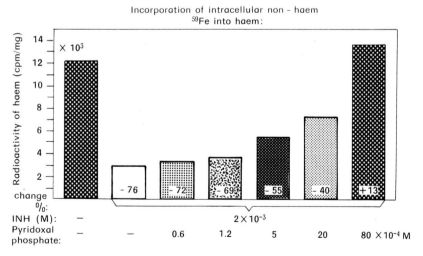

Fig. 15. The effect of various concentrations of pyridoxal phosphate on the incorporation of radioiron into haem and reticulocytes incubated with INH. (From *Poňka* and *Neuwirt*, 1971b.)

that by this interference with intracellular iron metabolism haem controls the overall rate of haem synthesis in erythroid cells. Evidence for this concept is presented in more detail elsewhere (p. 82).

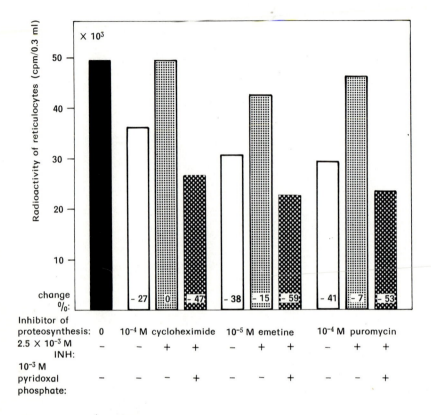

Fig. 16. The effect of inhibitors of globin synthesis on ^{59}Fe uptake by reticulocytes with inhibited (samples incubated with added INH) or restored (INH added together with pyridoxal phosphate) haem synthesis (From *Poňka* and *Neuwirt*, 1971b.)

Recent experiments concerning the influence of haem and inhibitors of haem and globin synthesis on the iron uptake by bone-marrow cells are of considerable importance (*Yamada et al.*, 1975; *Neuwirt* and *Poňka*, unpublished). The results of these experiments (Table 2) indicate that at the level of nucleated erythroid cells of bone marrow the iron uptake is also controlled by the negative feedback inhibition due to haem.

44

Table 2

The effect of various inhibitors on marrow cell uptake of transferrin bound ^{59}Fe and its incorporation into haem

Addition	Conc. (M)	Incorporation of ^{59}Fe into	
		Cells	Haem
Control		100	100
Haemin	$4 \cdot 10^{-5}$	91	100
Haemin	$8 \cdot 10^{-5}$	72	84
Haemin	$1.6 \cdot 10^{-4}$	64	66
Cycloheximide	$8 \cdot 10^{-4}$	91 (100)*	–
Cycloheximide	$8 \cdot 10^{-4}$		
+ INH	$4 \cdot 10^{-3}$	106 (116)*	19

The results are expressed as percentages of ^{59}Fe-incorporation into control bone-marrow cells or into *cycloheximide-incubated bone-marrow cells (*Poňka* and *Neuwirt*, unpublished).

Mechanism of the effect of haem on iron uptake

Recent experiments provide some insight into the mechanism of haem action (*Poňka et al.*, 1974, 1975; *Neuwirt et al.*, 1975a; *Schulman et al.*, 1974; *Fielding* and *Speyer*, 1974; *Poňka* and *Neuwirt*, 1975a). Haem does not block the uptake of the transferrin−iron complex, on the contrary in the presence of haem the amount of labelled transferrin molecules in reticulocytes increases (Fig. 17). All further experiments quoted below support the idea that haem inhibits the process of iron release from transferrin (*see* Fig. 31, p. 81).

Morgan (1971) described a simple method for the investigation of the rate of iron release from transferrin. The principle of the method is the ability of bipyridine to bind bivalent iron which is released from transferrin in the presence of reticulocytes. Bipyridine with bound iron leaves the cell and the amount of ^{59}Fe transferred to bipyridine can be taken as a measure of dissociation of iron from transferrin. Table 3 shows that the rate of iron exchange between transferrin and bipyridine in the presence of reticulocytes is markedly inhibited by haemin. Moreover, a similar but less significant inhibition was observed in the presence of cycloheximide which elevates the intracellular non-haemoglobin haem pool. This effect of cycloheximide can be prevented by addition of an inhibitor of haem synthesis (INH) (*Poňka et al.*, 1974).

In the presence of haem the relative amount of low-molecular iron (induced by

45

INH) declines and the incorporation of ^{59}Fe into haem from transferrin-^{59}Fe associated with reticulocytes is inhibited (*Poňka et al.*, 1974). Haem reduces the utilization of citrate-bound ^{59}Fe for haem synthesis (*Poňka*, unpublished data) whereby it is

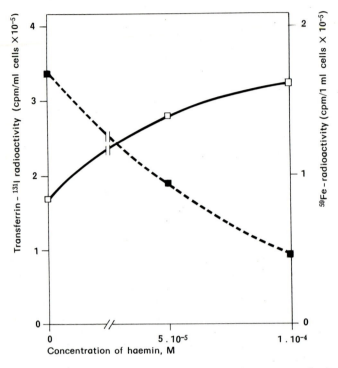

Fig. 17. Effect of haemin on the distribution of human transferrin-^{131}I and ^{59}Fe in reticulocytes after a 5-min incubation. Reticulocytes (0.5 ml) were incubated in the standard incubation medium with human transferrin-^{131}I or transferrin-^{59}Fe in a total volume of 1.5 ml. Both labelled transferrins were 50% saturated with cold iron. The cells were washed 4 times with cold saline solution, and the radioactivity of ^{131}I and ^{59}Fe of cells was counted. Radioactivity: □ = transferrin-^{131}I; ■ = ^{59}Fe. (From *Poňka et al.*, 1974. Reproduced with the permission of S. Karger AG, Basle.)

known that citrate-bound ^{59}Fe is incorporated into haem via transferrin present in reticulocytes. These results provide further evidence for the idea that haem inhibits the release of iron from transferrin. The finding of the inhibitory effect of haem on the pathway of iron from the transferrin — receptor site complex also confirms the above conclusion (*Fielding* and *Speyer*, 1975). If iron is released from transferrin on mitochondria, then the accumulation of transferrin-^{131}I in mitochondria isolated from haem-treated reticulocytes (Table 4) (*Neuwirt et al.*, 1975) can be explained on the basis of the above results.

46

Table 3

Effect of various inhibitors on uptake of transferrin-bound iron by reticulocytes and exchange of iron between transferrin and bipyridine in the presence of reticulocytes*

Additions	Iron uptake µg/h/ml reticulocytes	Control %	Iron transfer to bipyridine µg/h/ml reticulocytes	Control %
Control	0.46	100.0	0.54	100.0
Cycloheximide (10^{-3}M)	0.43	93.4	0.42	77.7
Cycloheximide (10^{-3}M) + INH (10^{-2}M)	0.51	110.8	0.51	94.4
Haemin (5×10^{-5}M)	0.32	69.5	0.31	57.4
Haemin (10^{-4}M)	0.16	34.7	0.16	29.6

*Reticulocytes (30% reticulocytosis) were incubated with purified human transferrin-^{59}Fe either alone (iron uptake) or with dialysis against 2mM 2,2'-bipyridine (iron transfer to bipyridine). Three samples were incubated in each group.
(From Poňka et al., 1974. Reproduced with the permission of S. Karger AK, Basle.)

Table 4

Distribution of human transferrin-^{131}I radioactivity in rabbit reticulocyte mitochondria and stroma-free supernatant. Effect of haemin

		Time of incubation (min)	Transferrin-^{131}I (cpm/ml cells)	Control (%)
Mitochondria	Control	0 20	5,960 22,871	100.0
	Haemin ($2 . 10^{-5}$M)	0 20	– 40,067	175.2
Stroma-free supernatant	Control	0 20	21,250 90,200	100.0
	Haemin ($2 . 10^{-5}$M)	0 20	– 225,096	249.5

(From Neuwirt et al., 1975a. Reproduced with the permission of Elsevier/North-Holland Biomedical Press B.V., Amsterdam.)

The increased amount of transferrin in reticulocytes during short-term incubation with haemin (Fig. 17, Table 4) is probably due to the fact that iron-transferrin molecules have a longer residence time on reticulocytes than iron-free transferrin molecules (*Baker* and *Morgan*, 1969b). In reticulocytes incubated with haem accumulation of iron-transferrin molecules, which are released slowly, may be expected. Actually the reduced release of transferrin from reticulocytes preincubated with haem has been demonstrated experimentally (Fig. 18) (*Poňka et al.*, 1975).

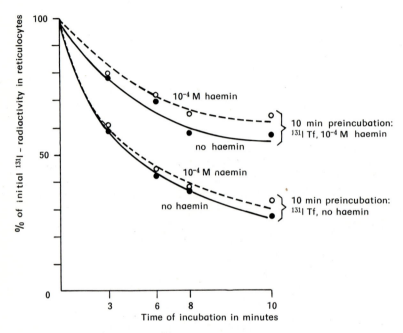

Fig. 18. Kinetics of release of transferrin-^{131}I (Tf) from reticulocytes. Effect of haemin. Rabbit reticulocytes (0.5 ml) were preincubated in the standard incubation mixture with human transferrin-^{131}I (50% saturated cold iron) in a total volume of 1.5 ml. Some samples were preincubated for 10 min with haemin, as indicated in the Figure. After preincubation with transferrin-^{131}I the cells were 4 times washed with cold saline to remove the label. The release of transferrin-^{131}I from cells was then studied. Reticulocytes were incubated in the standard incubation mixture with non-labelled human transferrin. Radioactivities of the cells and supernatants were counted. (From *Poňka et al.*, 1975. Reproduced with the permission of University of Tokyo Press, Tokyo.)

So far it is not possible to explain exactly the mechanism by which haem interferes with the process of iron dissociation from transferrin. It seems that haem does not interfere directly with the iron—transferrin complex (*Borová* and *Poňka*, unpublished data). Haem, which is known to inhibit various mitochondrial enzymes, incl. NADH-cytochrome-c reductase (*Silverstein*, 1962), might act as an inhibitor of the transfer of electrons in the respiratory chain. It has been mentioned already that the intact flow of electrons is essential for the release of iron from transferrin (p. 22).

It is, however, also important to consider the alternative possibility which is based on the observation that haem inhibits the release of bicarbonate from transferrin in the presence of reticulocytes (*Schulman et al.*, 1974; *Poňka et al.*, 1975) (Fig. 19). The dissociation of iron from transferrin probably depends on the enzymatic removal of bicarbonate from transferrin (p. 22) and haem might inhibit the enzyme respon-

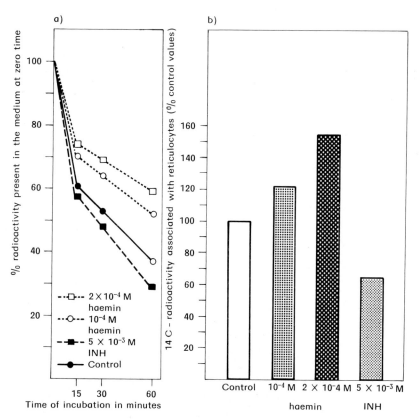

Fig. 19. The effect of haemin or INH on the release of bicarbonate-^{14}C from transferrin in the presence of reticulocytes (a) and on the uptake of bicarbonate-^{14}C-transferrin by reticulocytes (b). 0.3 ml of reticulocytes were incubated at 37 °C in a total volume of 1 ml incubation mixture. The concentration of transferrin (purified human, Behringwerke) was 0.51 mg per ml of media. Transferrin was labelled with H^{14}CO$_3^-$. At indicated time intervals the samples were withdrawn and placed in an ice-cold bath. The supernatant was removed after centrifugation and 100 μl of supernanant were dried and assayed for radioactivity. Four-times washed reticulocytes, taken after 60 minutes of incubation, were haemolyzed in 0.7 ml of distilled H$_2$O, then additional 4.0 ml of H$_2$O were added and 100 μl of haemolysate were dried and assayed for radioactivity. (From *Poňka et al.*, 1975. Reproduced with the permission of University of Tokyo Press, Tokyo.)

sible for the enzymatic attack on bicarbonate. This inhibition could be due to a reduced concentration of cyclic AMP in the excess haem, as inhibition of iron incorporation into reticulocytes caused by haem can be prevented by addition of dibutyryl cyclic AMP to the incubation medium (Table 5). Haem might exert its effect by reducing the concentration of cyclic AMP in reticulocytes; consequently the enzyme splitting off bicarbonate from transferrin is less activated and thus the rate of iron release from transferrin declines (*Poňka* and *Neuwirt*, 1975a). Before this hypothesis is accepted, it is, however, necessary to provide direct evidence that haem actually changes the level of cyclic AMP in erythroid cells.

Table 5

Effect of dibutyryl cyclic AMP (db-cAMP) on iron (bound to transferrin) incorporation into reticulocytes incubated with haemin. The results are expressed as percentages of controls

Haemin conc. (M)	Concentration of db-cAMP (M)				
	0	10^{-4}	$5 . 10^{-4}$	10^{-3}	$2 . 10^{-3}$
$5 . 10^{-6}$	95.1		111.8	113.6	
10^{-5}	78.1	84.2	95.6		
10^{-5}	94.9			108.2	
10^{-5}	94.9		87.5*	85.0*	
10^{-5}	82.8			102.9	
$1.25 . 10^{-5}$	92.7**		100.4**	103.0**	
$2 . 10^{-5}$	76.6			89.7	
$2 . 10^{-5}$	76.6		73.5*	68.5*	
$5 . 10^{-5}$	45.0			58.1	59.1

* 5-AMP (in indicated conc.) was added instead of db-cAMP.
** plasma-^{59}Fe was added instead of transferrin-^{59}Fe.
(From *Poňka* and *Neuwirt*, 1975a. Reproduced with the permission of Elsevier/North-Holland Biomedical Press B.V., Amsterdam.)

REGULATION OF UPTAKE OF GLYCINE AND OTHER AMINO ACIDS

There are two sources of amino acids for haemoglobin synthesis in immature erythroid precursors. Reticulocytes are above all known to concentrate various amino acids by transport systems which are not present in mature erythrocytes (*Riggs et al.*, 1952; *Allen*, 1960; *Winter* and *Christensen*, 1965; *Yunis* and *Arimura*, 1965; *Antonioli* and *Christensen*, 1969). In addition to the supply of amino acids from exogenous sources, amino acids are probably also released from endogenous sources in the reticulocyte. During reticulocyte maturation proteins of the stroma are broken down and the released amino acids can be utilized for haemoglobin synthesis (*Schweiger*, 1962).

From the point of view of haemoglobin synthesis, studies pertaining to amino acid transport during reticulocyte maturation when haemoglobin synthesis declines gradually, are most important. Of equal importance are investigations of the effect of metabolic inhibitors, in particular of protein synthesis, on the rate of amino acid uptake by reticulocytes. In 1952 *Riggs et al.* provided evidence that during reticulocyte maturation the ability to concentrate glycine and alanine disappears and at the same time the sensitivity of transport of these amino acids to dinitrophenol, cyanide (*cf. also* Fig. 21) and arsenate declines. Further investigations by *Christensen et al.* revealed that during maturation at least two Na^+-dependent transport systems are lost. The reduced glycine uptake after maturing does not result from a quantitative decline in the intensity of all transport systems but from the diminution of two transport systems beyond experimental detectability, while a further system remains intact (*Winter* and *Christensen*, 1965). During reticulocyte maturation the transport of other amino acids also declines (*Antonioli* and *Christensen*, 1969).

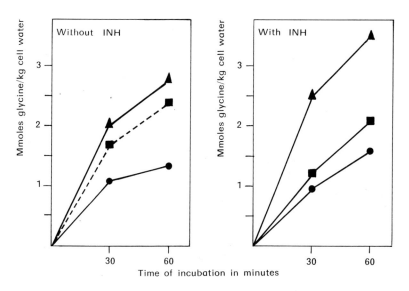

Fig. 20. The effect of haemin on glycine-2-^{14}C uptake by reticulocytes with normal or inhibited haem synthesis by INH (5 mM). The final concentration of glycine in the incubation mixture was 3.3 mM. Each value is the mean of three samples. —▲—, control; ---■---, 0.05 mM haemin; —○—, 0.1 mM haemin. (From *Neuwirt* and *Poňka*, 1972. Reproduced with the permission of J. F. Lehmanns Verlag, Munich.)

51

Some authors tried to find out whether changes in amino acid transport are related in any way to the declining protein synthesis. It was, however, shown that puromycin which completely inhibited protein synthesis did not influence the uptake of alanine and lysine by reticulocytes (*Yunis* and *Arimura*, 1965; *Wheeler* and *Christensen*, 1967) and similarly cycloheximide does not reduce the transport of leucine, methionine and phenylalanine (*Neuwirt* and *Poňka*, 1972 and unpublished results). Differences in amino acid transport by erythroid cells of different age thus cannot be explained by a different rate of protein synthesis.

Recently evidence was provided that haemin added to reticulocytes incubated *in vitro* inhibits the glycine uptake by these cells (*Neuwirt* and *Poňka*, 1972). The effect of haemin is obviously specific for transport systems for glycine and serine because of all investigated amino acids (glycine, serine, leucine, valine, methionine, phenylalanine and glutamic acid) only the transport of glycine and to a smaller extent that of serine is significantly inhibited. In this connection it is relevant to mention the finding of *Iyer* (1968) who observed that iron deficient erythrocytes take up markedly more glycine than normal erythrocytes. Similarly erythrocytes of patients with sideroblastic anaemias have significantly raised glycine concentrations (*Seip et al.*, 1971). Haem synthesis in iron deficient erythroid cells and in erythroblasts

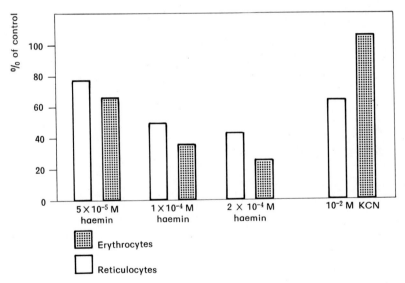

Fig. 21. The effect of haemin and cyanide on glycine-2-^{14}C uptake into reticulocytes and erythro-cytes. Reticulocytosis was induced by repeated bleeding. Reticulocyte-free erythrocytes were obtained from whole-body irradiated rabbits (5 days after 600 R). The results are expressed as per cent of control glycine uptake (i.e. without haemin or KCN) by red cells. The uptake of glycine into erythrocytes was 47 per cent of glycine uptake by reticulocyte-rich red blood cells (about 15 per cent reticulocytes). (*Poňka* and *Neuwirt*, unpublished.)

52

of patients with sideroblastic anaemias is evidently reduced. We provided evidence that haemin inhibits glycine transport in control reticulocytes as well as in cells incubated with INH which inhibits haem synthesis (Fig. 20). It is of interest that glycine transport is always more markedly inhibited in mature erythrocytes than in reticulocytes (Fig. 21). Therefore it seems that haemin inhibits only or mainly the transport systems for glycine that persist at the stage of mature erythrocytes. The experiment illustrated in Fig. 22 shows that the inhibitory effect of haemin on glycine transport depends only to a minor extent on the rate of protein synthesis in reticulocytes. This figure indicates moreover that haemin probably stimulates the incorporation of some amino acids into the free intracellular pool.

From these results it cannot so far be concluded whether the effect of haemin on amino acid transport can be reflected in some way in the regulation of haemo-

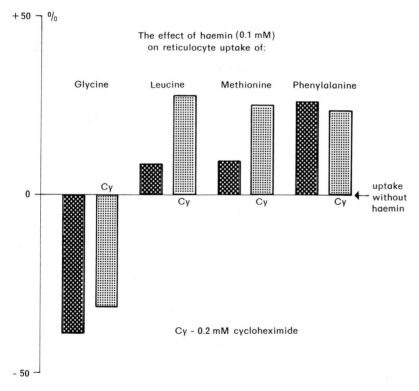

Fig. 22. The change in the uptake of various amino acids caused by haemin added to reticulocytes with normal or by cycloheximide inhibited globin synthesis. The results are expressed as difference (per cent) from the uptake without added haemin. Each value is based on values from two estimations. (From *Neuwirt* and *Poňka*, 1972. Reproduced with the permission of J. F. Lehmanns Verlag, Munich.)

53

globin synthesis. The results, however, suggest the complex role of haem in the metabolism of erythroid cells.

The observed effect of haem on glycine transport **provides** evidence of another feedback inhibition of substrate transport by the end product (cf. p. 82). This type of regulation may be of general importance as feedback regulation — mediated by the metabolic derivative of the substrate — was also described in other transport systems (for reference *see Ring et al.*, 1970).

The above results are also of certain importance from the methodological aspect. Interference of haemin with glycine uptake by reticulocytes must also be considered in experiments where labelled glycine is used for investigations of the effect of haemin on haemoglobin synthesis. The difference in the extent of stimulation of leucine and glycine incorporation into globin observed in some experiments (*see* Table 13, *Poňka et al.*, 1970) can be explained by the effect of haemin on the membrane transport of glycine.

3. HAEM SYNTHESIS

BIOSYNTHESIS OF HAEM

GENERAL INTRODUCTION

All aerobic cells, bacterial, plant and animal are able to synthesize haem. In the present chapter the most important aspects of haem synthesis in erythroid cells are discussed.

Our first knowledge of porphyrin synthesis dates back to 1946 when *Shemin* and *Ritternberg* published their classical work where, using labelled substances, they were able to determine the course of the initial stages of porphyrin synthesis. Investigations in *Shemin's* and *Neuberger's* laboratory revealed that all carbon and nitrogen atoms in haem are provided by glycine and succinate.

Porphyrin synthesis starts by condensation of the complex: glycine and pyridoxal phosphate with succinyl-CoA. Condensation of glycine and succinyl-CoA to δ-amino-laevulinic acid (ALA) is catalyzed by δ-aminolaevulinic acid synthetase (ALA synthetase) which is an enzyme which needs pyridoxal phosphate for its action. In the first stage of this reaction α-amino-β-oxoadipic acid is formed which is gradually decarboxylated to ALA. Two molecules of ALA are condensed with the participation of ALA dehydrase and monopyrrole, porphobilinogen (PBG) is formed.

Synthesis of the δ-aminolaevulinic acid is the first controlled stage in the series of reactions leading to porphyrin synthesis, while pyrrole synthesis is the stage where aromatization occurs. These two reactions of porphyrin metabolism may be controlled by end-product feedback inhibition or feedback repression. In the majority of systems studied it was revealed that the limiting factor of porphyrin synthesis is ALA synthesis.

In the presence of two enzymes — porphobilinogen deaminase and uroporphyrinogen III-cosynthetase — four molecules are gradually combined and they form a large circular colourless tetrapyrrole, uroporphyrinogen. Because substitution by two side-chains, acetate and propionate, is possible on two β-carbon atoms of phorphobilinogen four different isomers of uroporphyrinogen are formed. Isomer I is formed by the action of PBG deaminase either in the absence of uroporphyrinogen III-co-synthetase or probably under conditions when increased amounts of porphyrinogen are formed as it is the case in erythropoietic protoporphyria.

In isomer I four PBG molecules form a completely symmetrical compound, in isomer III two propionate side-chains are adjacent to two acetate side-chains. In nature only isomers I and III are found. In haem, chlorophyll and vitamin B_{12} only isomer III is present.

In the next stage by gradual decarboxylation of four acetate side-chains copropor-phyrinogen III is formed.

For the next reaction oxygen is needed which oxidizes two propionate chains in the presence of coproporphyrinogen oxidase. Propionate chains are converted to vinyl groups and a colourless molecule, protoporphyrinogen IX is formed. Protopor-phyrinogen IX is transformed by auto-oxidation and loss of hydrogen atoms to protoporphyrin which is bright red.

With protoporphyrin IX iron combines to form haem. This reaction is catalyzed by the enzyme called haem synthetase or ferrochelatase.

According to all contemporary knowledge the biosynthesis of porphyrin described above is used by all forms of life to produce haem or chlorophyll (Figs. 23 and 24).

It seems that in later stages of porphyrin synthesis the presence of a low-molecular co-factor is not necessary. It is also interesting that in these reactions phosphorylated intermediary products do not participate. It may be assumed that after formation of ALA a major energy expenditure is no longer needed for further metabolic reactions of porphyrin synthesis although the energetics of individual reactions have not been accurately assessed so far.

The presence of oxygen is needed at two sites. The first point is citrate oxidation

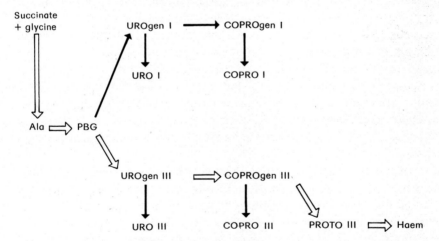

Fig. 23. Biosynthesis of haem. ALA, δ-aminolaevulinic acid; PBG, porphobilinogen; UROgen, uroporphyrinogen, COPROgen, coproporphyrinogen; URO, uroporphyrin; COPRO, copro-porphyrin; PROTO, protoporphyrin. (From *Scholnick et al.*, 1971. Reproduced with permission of the authors and the Rockefeller University Press, New York.)

in the Krebs cycle which is necessary for the formation of succinyl-CoA. The second point is the oxidation of coproporphyrinogen to protoporphyrinogen.

All erythroid cells with the exception of mature erythrocytes synthesize haem. The initiation of haemoglobin synthesis in erythroid precursor cells is associated with an increased formation of ALA synthetase. During maturation the limiting effect of different enzymes changes. Reticulocytes still contain remnants of mitochondria and synthesize uroporphyrin, coproporphyrin and protoporphyrin and

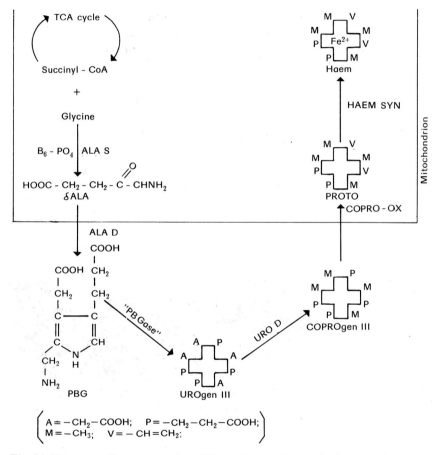

Fig. 24. Diagrammatic representation of the major steps in porphyrin biosynthesis. TCA cycle, tricarboxylic acid cycle; B_6-PO_4, pyridoxal phosphate; ALA S, ALA synthetase; ALA D, ALA dehydrase; "PBGase", is a term used to represent the enzymatic activity involved in the conversion of PBG to UROgen III. Two enzymes are actually involved in this conversion, PBG deaminase and an isomerizing enzyme; URO D, UROgen decarboxylase; COPRO-OX, COPROgen oxidase; HEME SYN, haem synthetase (ferrochelatase). Enzymes represented within the rectangle are located within mitochondria. (From *Perlroth et al.*, 1966. Reproduced with the permission of authors and Dun-Donnelley Publishing Corporation, New York.)

haem at a rate which declines progressively, depending on the gradual loss of mitochondrial ALA synthetase and haem synthetase. Enzymes required for the transformation of ALA to protoporphyrin disappear much more slowly and mature red cells are able to synthesize uroporphyrin and coproporphyrin from labelled ALA. Porphyrin synthesis from labelled glycine, as in haem synthesis, is, however, defective in these cells because for these reactions mitochondrial enzymes — ALA synthetase and haem synthetase — are needed.

Since 1948 it has been known that haem synthesis takes place *in vitro* in nucleated duck erythroid cells (*Shemin et al.*, 1948) and in anucleated rabbit reticulocytes (*London et al.*, 1950). Since then haem synthesis was commonly studied in avian red cells which resemble late mammalian erythroblasts as both these types of cells contain a nucleus and mitochondria and form haemoglobin. In chick erythrocytes incubated with glycine under aerobic conditions at 37°C haem and porphyrin syntheses take place at a constant rate for 24 hours (*Dresel* and *Falk*, 1956). *Dresel* and *Falk* calculated that this rate is four times slower than under conditions *in vivo*. In reticulocytes incubated *in vitro* haem synthesis stops much sooner.

After haemolysis of chick erythrocytes or reticulocytes porphyrin synthesis is greatly inhibited. It was shown that conversion of succinate and glycine to porphyrin can take place only in those cells which were very carefully haemolyzed with water (*Shemin* and *Russel*, 1954). On the other hand, the transformation of ALA to protoporphyrin IX is possible in homogenized preparations of avian erythrocytes as well as in a cell-free extract.

Haemoglobin synthesis was demonstrated also in nuclei of avian red cells (*Hammel* and *Bessman*, 1964). So far it is not quite clear whether enzymes of haem synthesis are present in these nuclei or whether haem penetrates into these nuclei from the cytoplasm.

Some enzymes of haem biosynthesis are soluble and after haemolysis of chick erythrocytes or rabbit reticulocytes they can be separated by starch electrophoresis (*Granick* and *Mauzerall*, 1958). Insoluble enzymes are present in mitochondria although their presence in nuclei cannot be quite ruled out. Soluble enzymes of haem biosynthesis include ALA dehydrase, PBG deaminase, uroporphyrinogen III-consynthetase and uroporphyrinogen decarboxylase. These enzymes are in the cytoplasm. ALA synthetase and the last two enzymes in the chain, coproporphyrinogen oxidase and haem synthetase, are mitochondrial enzymes.

It seems that mitochondrial enzymes are synthesized in ribosomes and then transported to mitochondria. *Kadenbach* (1970) demonstrated that apocytochrome-c from rat liver is synthesized in microsomes and then transported to mitochondria where it is joined by a haem group and holoenzyme is formed. It may be assumed that ferrochelatase and ALA synthetase are synthesized outside mitochondria and *Hayashi et al.* (1969, 1970) provided evidence that in the livers of porphyric rats ALA synthetase is also present in the cytoplasm. *Scholnick et al.* (1969) also detected soluble

58

ALA synthetase in normal rat liver and assumed that this soluble ALA synthetase is an enzyme on the pathway from ribosomes to mitochondria.

ALA SYNTHESIS

Shemin's investigations provided evidence that ALA is the first product in porphyrin biosynthesis and that it is formed from succinyl-CoA and glycine. The enzyme catalyzing this reaction, ALA synthetase, is generally considered the limiting stage of porphyrin biosynthesis. During ALA formation the complex of glycine and pyridoxal phosphate condenses with the carbonyl atom of succinyl-CoA (*Kikuchi et al.,* 1958; *Neuberger,* 1961) and α-amino-β-oxoadipic acid is formed. The latter is immediately decarboxylated and it is not clear whether it is present as an intermediary product bound to an enzyme or in the free form (Fig. 25). It is even possible that it is not an intermediary product at all as it cannot be ruled out that condensation and decarboxylation take place concurrently (*Tait,* 1968).

Investigations by *Lascelles* (1957) on *Tetrahymena vorax* confirmed that pyridoxal phosphate and coenzyme A are needed for this condensation. In the same year

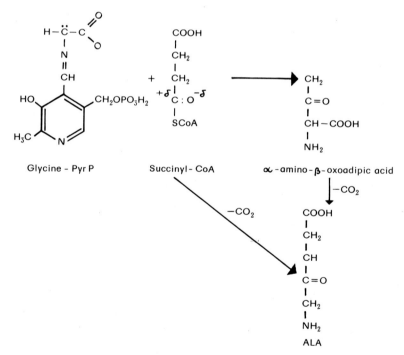

Fig. 25. Proposed mechanism of formation of ALA. (Taken from *Tait,* 1968. Reproduced with the permission of the author and the Biochemical Society, London.)

59

Schulman and *Richert* (1957) proved that pyridoxal phosphate restores haem synthesis in ducks with vitamin B_6 and pantothenic acid deficiency. *Granick* (1958) using pyridoxal phosphate inhibitors confirmed that for ALA synthesis the availability of pyridoxal phosphate is essential.

Gibson et al. (1958) were the first to prove that succinyl-CoA is one of the substrates for ALA synthetase. Succinyl-CoA can be formed by several metabolic pathways (*Granick* and *Levere*, 1964; *Mauzerall*, 1964). It was shown that sources of succinyl-CoA differ in animals and plants. In erythroid cells the main metabolic pathway which forms succinyl-CoA is oxidation of α-ketoglutaric acid by means of α-ketoglutarate oxidase, an enzyme localized in mitochondria.

On the other hand, in bacteria succinyl-CoA is formed from succinate, coenzyme A and ATP in the presence of Mg^{2+} ions by the enzyme succinyl-CoA synthetase (*Burnham*, 1963).

Shemin and *Kumin* (1952) concluded, based on their experiments with duck erythrocytes, that 30–50% succinyl-CoA can be derived directly from added succinate. In liver mitochondria from porphyric animals it was shown that after intoxication of mitochondria with arsenic compounds, when glycine and α-ketoglutarate are used as substrates, the formation of succinyl-CoA is reduced by 85%. From this ensues that only 15% succinyl-CoA is formed directly from succinate by the action of succinyl-CoA synthetase, while the remaining 85% is derived from the oxidation of α-ketoglutarate (*Granick* and *Levere*, 1964).

Two other possible ways of succinyl-CoA synthesis are its formation from propionyl-CoA which is a metabolic pathway important for sheep and ruminants and finally synthesis from acetyl-CoA to succinate by means of CoA transferase. So far it is not clear whether these two metabolic pathways are of any importance in erythroid cells (*Granick* and *Levere*, 1964).

Some experiments revealed that substances which cause an increased porphyrin formation inhibit NADH oxidase. This finding led to the assumption that inhibition of terminal oxidation is an important factor in the control of porphyrin and haem synthesis (*Labbe*, 1967; *Labbe et al.*, 1969, 1970). *Labbe et al.* proposed that porphyrogenic substances act on the redox potential of mitochondria and induce NAD-dependent reduction of fumarate with formation of succinate. Succinate then induces succinyl-CoA synthetase and the succinyl-CoA formed induces ALA synthetase by substrate induction. *Gajdos* and *Gajdos-Török* (1969) provided evidence that already before the increased activity of ALA synthetase the NADH concentration in the liver rises. It was therefore assumed that the ratio NADH-NAD is important for the regulation of porphyrin synthesis. *Labbe et al.* (1970) demonstrated that NAD suppressed the induction of ALA synthetase by substances producing porphyrin.

Gajdos and *Gajdos-Török* (1969) maintain, however, that before increased porphyrin formation the NADH concentration is increased but they emphasize at the same time that after 3 hours there is no longer any relationship between the rate of

60

porphyrin formation and NADH concentration. These workers tried to prove that the ATP concentration is one of the decisive factors in porphyrinogenesis. The lower the ATP concentration, the higher according to *Gajdos* and *Gajdos-Török* is porphyrin synthesis and ALA synthetase activity. It is assumed that administration of ATP or its high concentration enhance glycine utilization for lipid synthesis and probably also succinate utilization for some intracellular compounds, and thus reduce the amount of these substances needed for porphyrin synthesis. It cannot be ruled out that ATP stimulates the production of the physiological inhibitor of porphyrin synthesis. *Gajdos* admits, however, that this postulated regulatory effect of ATP does not fit our present knowledge of porphyrin synthesis. *Pinelli* and *Capuano* (1973) provide evidence that the reduction of ATP after administration of porphyrinogenic substances is associated with a reduction of the cAMP level. Low cAMP levels in cells are always associated with an increased ALA synthetase activity, while administration of dibutyryl cAMP reduces porphyrin production. On the other hand it must be mentioned that in tissue cultures of human foetal livers (*Congote et al.*, 1974) and bone marrow cells from normal non-porphyric animals (*Brown* and *Adamson*, 1974) cAMP stimulates ALA synthetase activity and haem synthesis (*Bottomley et al.*, 1971).

ALA SYNTHETASE

ALA synthetase is a universally occurring enzyme but so far it has been found in only a relatively small number of cells. It is generally assumed that ALA synthetase is the limiting stage of porphyrin synthesis and thus cells which form only a small amount of haem or vitamin B_{12} produce only small amounts of this enzyme. The highest activities of ALA synthetase were found in photosynthetic bacteria which grow rapidly and have a high content of bacteriochlorophyll and haem proteins. Avian and mammalian reticulocytes where haemoglobin synthesis takes place, also have a relatively high activity. In a number of cellular systems the activity of ALA synthetase is markedly raised when the cells are exposed to the action of inducing porphyrinogenic substances which enhance porphyrin synthesis.

The fact that it is impossible to detect ALA synthesis in the majority of tissues is explained by some workers by the presence of an ubiquitous inhibitor. This inhibitor was also found in liver extracts, extracts from avian erythrocytes, photosynthetic bacteria and some other sources (*Shemin*, 1970). In *Rhodopseudomonas spheroides* ALA synthetase is activated by addition of cystine (*Neuberger et al.*, 1973). It was revealed that in particular cystine trisulfide is active and increases the enzyme activity as much as seven times. *Tuboi* and *Hayasaka* (1973) maintain that in *Rhodopseudomonas spheroides* ALA synthetase is present in two fractions. Both fractions, I and II, can exist either in the active or inactive form. The transformation from the active to

61

the inactive form takes place in particular in the presence of sulfhydryl substances, e.g. L-cystein. The mechanism of transformation of the active into the inactive form probably involves a sulfhydryl-disulfide exchange.

ALA synthetase has not been prepared so far in pure form although reports from some laboratories speak of a considerable degree of purification (*Kikuchi et al.*, 1958; *Burnham* and *Lascell*, 1963; *Scholnick et al.*, 1969; *Bottomley*, 1969; *Aoki et al.*, 1971).

Bottomley and *Smithee* (1968) proved ALA synthetase in normal rabbit bone marrow and assessed its activity in mitochondria of cells broken by sonication.

Optimal conditions for the assessment of ALA synthetase in mitochondria of rabbit bone marrow are very similar to those for the enzyme of avian erythrocytes, in particular with regard to the optimum pH and optimum glycine and α-keto-glutarate concentration in the incubation medium (*Laver et al.*, 1958; *Brown*, 1958; *Gibson et al.*, 1958). It was revealed that in bone marrow ALA synthetase can be quantitatively assessed although it must be realized that ALA synthesis also takes place in mitochondria of cells other than erythroid. It may, however, be assumed that almost all estimated ALA comes from erythroid cells as the amount of haem needed for haemoglobin synthesis is incomparably greater than the minimum amount of haem needed for the synthesis of the other haem enzymes.

Feldman and *Lichtman* (1967) measured the ALA synthetase activity in normal human reticulocytes. Insoluble particles containing mitochondria were obtained from the haemolysate of peripheral blood by the method of *Laver et al.* (1957).

Bottomley and *Smithee* (1969) described the isolation of partly purified ALA synthetase from rabbit bone marrow and assessed its properties. The enzyme was purified 300 times and solubilization of isolated mitochondria with sodium cholate, sequence chromatography on Sephadex G-200, Biogel A and hydroxylapatite was used for this purpose. The purified enzyme on disc gel electrophoresis was separated into two bands and was stable at 4°C for 48 hours. The molecular weight was about 300,000 daltons (measured by gel filtration) and the maximum absorption occurred at 260 nm. The enzymatic properties recalled the properties of a mitochondrial preparation except that the constant for glycine was 1×10^{-3} M. Haem inhibits this partly purified enzyme already at a concentration of 1×10^{-5} M.

Aoki et al. (1971) isolated ALA synthetase from rabbit reticulocytes and were able to increase its activity about 4400 times. The purified enzyme was homogeneous when subjected to disc gel electrophoresis. The optimum pH was 7.6 and the iso-electric point 5.9. For the action of the enzyme the presence of pyridoxal phosphate was necessary. Haem inhibited the activity of the purified enzyme in a concentration of 1×10^{-5} M to an extent of about 40%. The K_m for succinyl CoA in this system is 6×10^{-5} M and for glycine 1×10^{-2} M. The molecular weight of the enzyme is cca 200,000 daltons according to its elution behaviour on a Sephadex G-200 column.

ALA synthetase is localized inside the matrix space of mitochondria (*McKay et al.*,

1969). *Zuyderhoudt et al.*, (1969) induced ALA synthetase synthesis in rats by means of allylisopropyl acetamide (AIA) and found that the enzyme is intramitochondrial. These experiments revealed that ALA synthetase is a matrix enzyme defined in the common sense of the word, i.e. either present in the free form in the matrix space or so loosely bound to the inner membrane that it is released by sonic fragmentation of mitochondria.

Hayaschi et al. (1969, 1970) and *Scholnick et al.* (1969) provided evidence that in rats after induction by AIA, ALA synthetase did not accumulate only in mitochondria but also in the cytoplasm. Soluble ALA synthetase increases about 10 times after administration of substances inducing porphyrin synthesis. This increase corresponds to the increase of ALA synthetase in mitochondria. In porphyric rats soluble ALA synthetase accounted for 40% of the entire ALA synthetase activity.

Kikuchi et al. (1975) found that ALA synthetase, the synthesis of which in animals is induced by allylisopropylacetamide, cumulates in the cytosol fraction. The molecular weight of this enzyme assessed by gel filtration is 600,000 daltons and assessed by gradient centrifuging 178,000 daltons. The mitochondrial enzyme, i.e. the enzyme isolated from mitochondria, has a molecular weight of 110,000 daltons measured by both methods. The authors conclude that cytosol ALA synthetase is a complex of ALA synthetase with a molecular weight of 110,000 daltons and some 4s protein. This complex gives aggregates with a molecular weight of 300,000 daltons or 600,000 daltons. Under physiological conditions the complex is then exposed to limited proteolysis, loses the ability to form aggregates and the enzyme with a molecular weight of 110,000 daltons is incorporated into mitochondria.

ALA synthetase in the cytoplasm is probably an enzyme on the path from ribosomes to mitochondria. This enzyme needs for its action the same substrates and cofactors as mitochondrial ALA synthetase.

This intracellular localization of ALA synthetase corresponds to the concept that enzymes formed on ribosomes of the endoplasmatic reticulum are transformed into the soluble form and travel to specific sites of destination in mitochondria. It is assumed that ALA synthetase is broken down only in the cytoplasm, while during the passage through mitochondria it is protected in some unknown way. According to these views ALA synthetase could enter mitochondria and leave them as well. *Hayashi et al.* (1969) confirmed that the half-life of the soluble enzyme is much shorter than the half-life of the mitochondrial enzyme.

ALA synthesis is significantly inhibited by aminomalonate and kinetic observation revealed that this inhibition is competitive in relation to glycine (*Gibson et al.*, 1961). Other inhibitors of ALA synthetase are ALA, 1-penicillamine, 1-cystine and cyanide ions. It is assumed that these inhibitors react directly with the aldehyde group of pyridoxal phosphate and thus form a thiazolidine ring or cyanohydrin (*Mauzerall*, 1964). It was shown that 1-penicillamine is an important antagonist of pyridoxal phosphate in biological systems (*Kuchinskas et al.*, 1957, *Ueda et al.*, 1960). In our own experiments isonicotinic acid hydrazide (INH) proved to be a potent inhibitor of ALA synthetase in rabbit reticulocytes.

90% of ALA added to haemolyzed chick erythrocytes are converted into porphyrins (*Dresel* and *Falk*, 1956). These results indicate that as soon as ALA is once formed in erythroid cells, only a small portion is oxidized. A small portion of ALA which is not utilized for porphyrin synthesis is metabolized in the so-called succinate-glycine cycle (*Shemin* and *Russel*, 1953). The quantitative importance of this cycle for ALA metabolism is so far not quite clear.

PORPHOBILINOGEN (PBG) SYNTHESIS. ALA DEHYDRASE ENZYME

By condensation of two ALA molecules the pyrrole porphobilinogen is formed and this reaction is catalyzed by the enzyme ALA dehydrase. Contrary to ALA synthetase, this enzyme is readily detected in extracts of the majority of animal plant and bacterial cells (*Gibson*, 1955).

ALA dehydrase was partly purified from rabbit reticulocytes (*Granick* and *Mauzerall*, 1958), human erythrocytes (*Calissano et al.*, 1966) and some other sources.

All enzymes obtained from various tissues are SH enzymes and their activity can be detected only after addition of SH substances. Heavy metals (e.g. lead) and substances reacting with sulfhydryls inhibit the activity of ALA dehydrase. To demonstrate the maximum activity of the enzyme most tissue extracts must be preincubated with thiols. This need of a highly reducing medium indicates that the oxidation-reduction potential of cells may play an important part in the control of the activity of this enzyme. When the oxidation-reduction potential is high, the enzyme activity is markedly reduced (*Tait*, 1968).

Inhibition of this enzyme by substances which are structurally related to ALA is very interesting, because of their possible use in preventing overproduction of porphyrins in porphyria. γ-aminoacetic acid, the lower homologue of ALA, is a mild inhibitor of the enzyme of chick erythrocytes and δ-oximinolaevulinic acid inhibits the liver enzyme of mice.

CONVERSION OF PORPHOBILINOGEN (PBG)
TO UROPORPHYRINOGEN III

The conversion of 4 molecules of PBG to tetrapyrrole uroporphyrinogen III requires two enzymes, uroporphyrinogen I synthetase (Fig. 26) (PBG deaminase) and uroporphyrinogen III co-synthetase (PBG isomerase). In the absence of the latter enzyme symmetrical uroporphyrinogen I is formed. The two enzymes mentioned have a different sensitivity to high temperature and this finding confirmed their existence. If the enzyme preparation is incubated with PBG, uroporphyrinogen III is formed. However, when cells containing uroporphyrinogen III co-synthetase are heated to 60°C for a period of 15 min, only uroporphyrinogen I is formed. This provides evidence that uroporphyrinogen III co-synthetase is sensitive to higher temperatures. *Booij* and *Rimington* (1957) demonstrated this phenomenon by preheating of red cells. Some time ago both enzymes were separated from mouse spleens (*Levin* and *Coleman*, 1967).

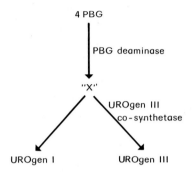

Fig. 26. The conversion of 4 PBG molecules into uroporphyrinogen III. (From *Tait*, 1968. Reproduced with the permission of the author and the Biochemical Society, London.)

PBG deaminase converts four molecules of PBG to uroporphyrinogen I by the following reaction:

$$4\,PBG \longrightarrow 1 \text{ uroporphyrinogen I} + 4\,NH_3$$

Under anaerobic conditions the yield of this reaction is almost 100%. This enzyme requires for its activity the presence of SH groups and acts only on PBG. The clue to the elucidation of mechanisms of uroporphyrinogen III formation is the identification of the substrate of uroporphyrinogen III co-synthetase. Exact mechanisms of biosynthesis of uroporphyrinogen III from PBG are far from clear. More than 20 hypotheses were presented on the transformation of porphobilinogens to uroporphyrinogens but none was confirmed. *Frydman et al.* (1973) studied this reaction intensively. They found that porphobilinogen is polymerized on the surface of the enzyme without releasing soluble intermediates (pyrryl methanes). During formation of uroporphyrinogen I two porphobilinogen units are condensed head to tail while by head-to-head condensation of the same units uroporphyrinogen III is formed. The formed dipyrryl methanes remain in all stages bound to the enzyme.

In erythropoietic porphyria isomeric type I uroporphyrins and coproporphyrins are formed in excess and are then excreted in the urine. This production of isomers I is explained as follows: PBG isomerase (uroporphyrinogen III co-synthetase) has for different reasons a low activity (*Booij* and *Rimington*, 1957; *Rimington* and *Booij*, 1957). It cannot be ruled out either that the isomerase activity may become limiting under conditions of excessive ALA production (*Granick* and *Levere*, 1964). It must be, however, emphasized that the preferential production of isomer III under normal conditions indicates that the degree of isomerization is not limiting.

CONVERSION OF UROPORPHYRINOGEN TO COPROPORPHYRINOGEN BY THE ENZYME UROPORPHYRINOGEN DECARBOXYLASE

The next stage in the biosynthesis of porphyrins is decarboxylation of four acetate side-chains of uroporphyrinogen with the formation of methyl groups, i.e. from porphyrinogen with eight carboxyl groups porphyrinogen with four of these groups is formed. The enzyme catalyzing the transformation of uroporphyrinogen to coproporphyrinogen III, uroporphyrinogen decarboxylase, was isolated from rabbit reticulocytes by means of starch gel electrophoresis (*Granick* and *Mauzerall*, 1958).

CONVERSION OF COPROPORPHYRINOGEN TO PROTOPORPHYRINOGEN BY THE ENZYME COPROPORPHYRINOGEN OXIDASE

The conversion of coproporphyrinogen III is catalyzed by coproporphyrinogen oxidase and this reaction comprises the decarboxylation and dehydrogenation of two propionate side-chains and two vinyl groups are formed. The product of this reaction is protoporphyrinogen which then loses its six hydrogen atoms to form a red coloured porphyrin. The enzyme mentioned is relatively specific for coproporphyrinogen III and does not act on isomers I and II. The formation of protoporphyrinogen from coproporphyrinogen was demonstrated in chick erythrocytes (*Granick* and *Mauzerall*, 1958) and in mitochondria of beef liver (*Granick* and *Sano*, 1961). Oxygen is the only oxidating agent which can be used by this enzyme.

COMBINATION OF IRON WITH PROTOPORPHYRIN

The combination of Fe^{2+} with protoporphyrin is catalyzed by the enzyme protohaemferrolyase which is better known by the name of ferrochelatase (*Rimington*, 1966), haem synthetase (*Riethmüller* and *Tuppy*, 1964) or haem synthase (*Porra* and *Ross*, 1965). During the combination of Fe^{2+} with various porphyrins two protons are released and the corresponding haems are formed.

Goldberg et al. (1956) were the first to show that the formation of haem from protoporphyrin and iron is an enzymatic reaction. Haem synthetase is a mitochondrial enzyme and has been detected in some animal tissues (*Krueger et al.*, 1956; *Schwartz et al.*, 1959; *Lockhead et al.*, 1963) and in microorganisms (*Porra* and *Jones*, 1963).

For haem formation only bivalent iron can be used and normal anaerobic con-

66

ditions are necessary. Trivalent iron Fe^{3+} can be used only when reducing agents are available and when the electron transport pathway is functional. *Jones* and *Jones* (1969) assumed that succinate oxidation reduces the oxygen concentration and thus prevents auto-oxidation of bivalent iron. The association of haem synthetase with electron transport in mitochondria is a mechanism by which the supply of bivalent iron from iron which is present in cells almost exclusively in the trivalent form is ensured. The oxygen concentration in the vicinity of mitochondria may be one of the factors which control haem synthesis. At high oxygen concentrations bivalent iron can be oxidized and the Fe^{2+} concentration does not reach the value of K_m (*Jones* and *Jones*, 1969). The high haem synthetase activity may, however, make it possible for haem to be formed even under these conditions.

Ascorbic acid increases the enzyme activity probably by stabilizing the enzyme by activation of its sulfhydryl groups. Ascorbic acid also participates, of course, in maintaining iron in the bivalent form. For enzyme activity in bone marrow and avian red cells the presence of glutathione is essential (*Bottomley*, 1968; *Goldberg et al.*, 1956).

Yoshikawa and *Yoneyama* (1964), *Mazanowska et al.* (1966) and *Tait* (1968) provided evidence that during iron incorporation into protoporphyrin an important part is played by some lipid. Fractionation of this lipid revealed that it is probably a phospholipid. Phosphatidyl ethanolamine and phosphatidyl choline do not influence incorporation, phosphatidylic acid, however, stimulates haem production as well as the formation of zinc protoporphyrin. *Yoshikawa* and *Yoneyama* (1964) described the inactivation of haem synthetase from the stroma of duck erythrocytes by phospholipase A. So far the role played by the lipid in the insertion of iron into the porphyrin is not clear.

Bottomley (1968) presented a report on the assessment of activity of haem synthetase in the lysate of human bone marrow prepared by successive freezing and thawing. The enzyme was sensitive to high temperatures and had an optimum pH of 7.4. K_m for iron was 1.7×10^{-5} and for protoporphyrin 0.18×10^{-5} M. The optimal protoporphyrin concentration for haem synthetase from bone marrow is very similar to the concentration which is optimal in avian erythrocytes (*Schwartz et al.*, 1959) and for the liver enzyme (*Labbe* and *Hubbard*, 1960). The activity of haem synthetase from human bone marrow increased after addition of ascorbic acid and glutathione (*Bottomley*, 1968).

Langelaan et al. (1969, 1970) found that the activity of haem synthetase can also be detected in fresh human blood. This activity is due to the presence of white cells and immature precursors of the erythroid series.

Haem synthetase has not yet been obtained in crystalline form. A partly purified preparation was achieved by *Yoneyama et al.* (1962) who were able to increase the activity of the enzyme of duck erythrocytes 200 times and by *Reitmüller* and *Tuppy* (1964) who increased the activity of the enzyme from yeast 70 times. *Mazanowska et al.* (1969) isolated haem synthetase from liver mitochondria by sonication and repeated freezing and thawing. After these procedures Tween 20 was added to mitochondria and the activity of the enzyme was increased 20 to 40 times by fractionation with ammonium sulphate and chromatography on dextran gel.

Lead inhibits the activity of haem synthetase. This effect together with the inhibition of ALA dehydrase by lead is the reason why lead poisoning is associated with reduced haemoglobin synthesis. Some other SH inhibitors inhibit haem synthetase activity as well.

Manyan and *Yunis* (1970) provided evidence that in dogs fed chloramphenicol, 100 mg/kg per day, the haem synthetase activity in bone marrow declined to 5–35% of control values. The effect of chloramphenicol was explained by inhibition of haem synthetase synthesis in mitochondria. Along with the decline of haem synthetase activity the level of free erythrocytic protoporphyrin and stainable iron in bone marrow increased considerably; these findings correspond to the block in the terminal stage of haem synthesis. Recently these workers (*Manyan et al.*, 1972) postulated the hypothesis that chloramphenicol may inhibit transport of enzymes from ribosomes into mitochondria.

The capacity of haem synthetase in liver mitochondria to synthesize protohaem is far higher than the activity needed for the biogenesis of haem in mitochondria (approximately 0.4 nmols/min/mg protein). Haem synthetase could produce the haem needed for mitochondria within a shorter period than three minutes and it would take a little longer before haem would be formed for extramitochondrial haemoproteins (*Jones* and *Jones*, 1969). The half-life of mitochondrial proteins is about 10 days. These figures indicate that in liver mitochondria haem synthetase cannot be the limiting enzyme. Unfortunately so far we do not possess similar data for erythroid cells.

FREE PROTOPORPHYRIN

Protoporphyrin is a red pigment present in traces in mature erythrocytes; reticulocytes and nucleated erythroid cells contain a little more. So far the role of protoporphyrin in erythroid cells has not yet been assessed. *Klein* presented the assumption (1968), based on his experiments with labelled glycine and protoporphyrin, that erythrocytes contain three protoporphyrin compartments. The first serves as the immediate source of porphyrin for haem and the second passes into plasma as a source of plasma porphyrins. The function of the third compartment is not clear although it seems that the porphyrin turnover in this compartment is very slow and that this part of the porphyrin is not immediately available for haem synthesis.

The amount of free erythrocytic protoporphyrin is influenced by many factors. The normal amount of protoporphyrin in red cells is 20–40 μg/100 ml and this amount may increase as much as ten times in iron deficiency anaemia and after haemorrhage.

All factors which increase the number of reticulocytes also increase the amount of free protoporphyrin. Its increase is also promoted by all conditions where iron incorporation into porphyrin is impaired. Erythrocytic protoporphyrin is reduced in pyridoxin deficiency, as this substance is needed as a co-factor for ALA synthetase.

REGULATION OF HAEM BIOSYNTHESIS

Investigations in aerobic bacteria and mammalian cells revealed that in these types of cells porphyrin and haem biosyntheses are regulated in a similar way. In all these aerobic cells the necessary enzymatic and structural conditions for haem formation obviously exist. In this connection it must be emphasized that all cells do not synthesize haem with equal intensity and in equal amounts. Erythroid cells contain 500–1000 times more haem than hepatocytes (*Kappas et al.*, 1968). It was revealed that rat bone marrow forms haem seven times more rapidly than rat liver (*Sassa* and *Granick*, 1970). This finding provides evidence that there are mechanisms in cells which ensure differentiated regulation of the activity of the haem synthetic chain.

Under physiological conditions the rate of haem synthesis is very closely associated with the coordination and rate of synthesis of different proteins. This mutual coordination of haem synthesis and the appropriate apoproteins is ensured by a number of very complicated mechanisms and feedbacks and will be discussed in detail in the chapter on regulation of haemoglobin synthesis.

Porphyrin and haem synthesis are controlled by the following mechanisms:

(1) Synthesis of enzymes of the porphyrin biosynthetic chain. This control can be effected either at the transcription or translation level.

(2) Changes in the activity of enzymes of the porphyrin biosynthetic chain.

(3) Supply of substrates needed for haem synthesis.

(4) Metabolic cytoplasmatic and external factors (e.g. oxygen tension, electron transport in the terminal chain, Krebs cycle, presence of SH substances, pyridoxal phosphate, etc.).

(5) Haem catabolism.

It is assumed that the enzyme limiting haem biosynthesis is the first enzyme of porphyrin biosynthesis, ALA synthetase. It seems that all the remaining enzymes are present in cells in non-limiting amounts. On the other hand it must be mentioned that some workers (*Calissano et al.*, 1966; *Bottomley*, 1968) assume that also other enzymes of porphyrin synthesis such as ALA dehydrase and haem synthetase can participate in the regulation of haem synthesis.

Mechanisms regulating haem synthesis will be now discussed in more detail.

ENZYME SYNTHESIS

Granick and *Urata* (1963) made a detailed investigation of enzymes involved in the biosynthesis of porphyrins in normal rat liver. The assessment of activity of all enzymes was relatively easy, only the activity of ALA synthetase could not be assessed. From this finding these authors concluded that porphyrin synthesis is limited by ALA synthetase. Further evidence for this statement was obtained in their subsequent experiments where they demonstrated that feeding guinea pigs on 3,5-dietoxycarbonyl-1,4-dihydro-2,4,6-trimethyl pyridine (DDC) caused overproduction of porphyrin and porphyrin precursors in the liver. This excessive porphyrin production was conditioned by a specific increase in ALA synthetase.

Incubation of mitochondria from normal guinea-pig livers with substances inducing enhanced porphyrin synthesis did not increase the activity of ALA synthetase. This indicates that the increase in ALA synthetase after administration of DDC is due to *de novo* synthesis of ALA synthetase and not to activation of the inactive enzyme. In his subsequent work *Garnick* (1966) demonstrated that the increase in ALA synthetase activity and increased porphyrin formation can be induced in livers from chick embryos *in vitro* by a number of substances. Experiments *in vitro* revealed also that substances which promote porphyrin synthesis act directly on liver tissue and not via hormones or some other factors.

Induction of ALA synthetase after administration of DDC can be almost completely prevented by mitomycin, actinomycin, puromycin and *p*-fluorophenylalanine (*Marver et al.*, 1966). Actinomycin blocks the formation of RNA and mitomycin causes depolymerization of DNA. Therefore it was concluded that for induction of ALA synthetase the presence of intact DNA is needed and that the increased activity of the enzyme results from its *de novo* synthesis. Isotope studies with labelled orotic acid and leucine revealed that addition of the inducing substance to liver cells did not lead to any changes in mRNA and protein synthesis (*Granick*, 1966). This shows that induction of synthesis of ALA synthetase is specific and does not apply to all proteins.

It was shown that a number of steroid derivatives formed by the biotransformation of C-19 and C-21 hormones (e.g. testosterone and progesterone) can induce increased porphyrin formation in very low concentrations (10^{-6} to 10^{-8} M). These steroid metabolites as regards their action equal or surpass the most potent porphyrinogens (*Granick* and *Kappas*, 1967). The most effective substances include etiocholanone, pregnandiole, 11-ketopregnanolone, pregnantriol, dehydroepiandrosterone and androstendione.

Formerly it was assumed that these substances are only inactive products of steroid metabolism *in vivo*. In erythroid cells ALA synthetase can be induced only by these 5-β-H steroids, while in chick embryo liver cells its formation can be induced by other substances and pharmaceutical preparations. Human liver does not respond to steroids in this way, mouse liver gives this response but must be stimulated concurrently by porphyrinogenic substances (*Weissman et al.*, 1973). These steroids are so far the only substances occurring under physiological conditions which influence porphyrin formation and it is therefore assumed that they participate actively in the control and regulation of haem synthesis (*Granick* and *Kappas*, 1967).

Patients with acute intermittent porphyria have a defect in the reductive transformation of steroid hormones. This defect is probably inherited, but it cannot be ruled out that some acquired factors also play their part. In this condition more 5-β-steroids are formed which induce ALA synthetase (*Kappas et al.*, 1972). Also oral contraceptives can cause porphyria (*Gajdos* and *Gajdos-Török*, 1973). Dihydroxycoprostan and trihydroxycoprostan, i.e. intermediary products in the synthesis of bile acids increase porphyrin synthesis in the liver. That these substances also have a physiological regulating effect on porphyrin synthesis cannot be excluded (*Javitt et al.*, 1973).

Granick (1966) expressed the hypothesis that the formation of ALA synthetase is controlled by a mechanism of feedback repression and that substances inducing porphyrin formation in some way eliminate this repressive control mechanism. According to this theory inducing substances replace haem (which acts as a co-repressor) by a competitive mechanism. When haem is replaced by inducing substances, more ALA synthetase is formed. This hypothesis is based on the findings of *Burnham* and *Lascelles* (1963) that haem represses ALA synthetase formation in *Rhodopseudomonas spheroides*. A theory has been submitted that the gene-regulator produces an aporepressor which after combination with haem (co-repressor) acts as a repressor on the gene-operator (Fig. 27). Substances which induce porphyrin formation prevent the combination of haem and the aporepressor, the gene operator is de-repressed and the code of the structural gene can be used for the production of ALA synthetase.

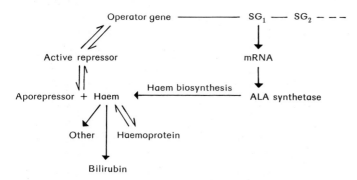

Fig. 27. Closed feedback representation of haem acting in the repression of ALA synthetase. SG, structural gene; mRNA, messenger RNA. (From *Waxman A. D. et al.*, 1966. Reproduced with the permission of the authors and Academic Press, Inc., New York.)

This hypothesis was tested by experiments to reveal competition between haem and allylisopropylacetamide (AIA) which is a substance inducing porphyrin formation.

Administration of substances which induce porphyrin formation reduces the haem and cytochrome P 450 concentration in liver microsomes (*Marver et al.*, 1968). The mechanism of this degradation of microsomal haem is so far not clear. These substances can either directly damage the haemoprotein molecule or haem only. The administration of some metals (Fe, Ni, Mn, Co, Cu, Zn) and heavy metals (Cd, Pb, Hg) also enhances microsomal haem degradation in liver cells and increases ALA synthetase activity. Simultaneously the haemoprotein content in microsomes declines by 40 to 60%. Increased oxidation of haem after administration of these metals was also found in other tissues. For instance a single injection of cobalt leads to a 50% increase in haem oxidation in the heart (*Maines* and *Kappas*, 1976). The probable relationship between an increased turnover of microsomal haem and induction of ALA synthetase was postulated in the work of *Meyer* and *Marver* (1971). The rapid turnover of microsomal haemoprotein may prevent haem from performing its normal repressor function.

Differences between induction of ALA synthetase formation by different substances in the liver and erythroid cells indicate that the increased formation of this enzyme may be brought about in two ways:

(1) by induction at the transcription level probably by influencing the synthesis of mRNA for ALA synthetase;

(2) by induction at the translation level, probably by influencing ALA synthetase synthesis (*Sassa* and *Granick*, 1970, 1971).

In chick embryo liver cells it was found that the half-life of mRNA for ALA synthetase is about 5 hours and the half-life of the enzyme is 3 hours (*Marver et al.*, 1966). Because mRNA has a relatively long half-life the effect of inducing substances on accumulation of mRNA can be studied during inhibition of protein synthesis by cycloheximide, or the synthesis of the enzyme can be studied from accumulated mRNA during inhibition of RNA synthesis by actinomycin D.

During inhibition of mRNA synthesis by actinomycin D AIA significantly increases the enzyme synthesis from preformed mRNA. AIA acts either by protracting the life span of mRNA for ALA synthetase or by increasing its translation activity.

Sassa and *Granick* (1970) provided evidence that there exist two types of inducing substances. One type (e.g. AIA) increases the activity of ALA synthetase in the presence of actinomycin D. The second type of inducing substances (e.g. etiocholanolone or DDC) does not increase the enzyme synthesis in the presence of actinomycin D. This latter group of inducing substances acts at the transcription level (Table 6).

Addition of haemin to a chick-embryo liver-cell culture inhibits synthesis of ALA synthetase. *Granick* (1966) expressed the hypothesis that haemin inhibits ALA synthetase synthesis at the transcription level (*see also* p. 71) but later evidence was provided (*Sassa* and *Granick*, 1970) that haemin inhibits ALA synthetase induction at the translation level. The cells in the culture were exposed for 14 hours to the action of AIA to increase the amount of ALA synthetase. The medium was then exchanged and replaced by a fresh medium with actinomycin D and haemin. It was revealed that the life span of ALA synthetase declined to 3.6 hours, a considerable reduction compared with 5.2 hours in the presence of actinomycin D only. This experiment provides evidence that haem inhibits ALA synthetase formation at the translation level.

Table 6

Controls on ALA synthetase at the transcriptional and translation levels

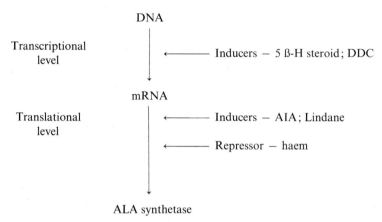

(From *Sassa* and *Granick*, 1970. Reproduced with the permission of authors and the National Academy of Sciences, Washington.)

Haem could act either by competition with inducing substances or reduce the life span of mRNA for ALA synthetase. This latter assumption, however, does not seem probable, as haem does not enhance ribonuclease activity. Haem also blocks the conversion of cytosol into mitochondrial ALA synthetase in porphyric animals.

Haematin administered by the i.v. route to patients with erythropoietic porphyria enters precursors in the bone marrow where it reduces the porphyrin concentration (*Watson et al.*, 1974).

As has been mentioned above, erythroid and chick-embryo hepatic tissues respond to induction by 5-β-H steroids by enhanced ALA synthetase formation. Induction by steroids in the liver takes place at the transcription level and it seems that in erythroid tissues also steroids induce enzyme synthesis at the transcription level. A number of substances and pharmaceutical preparations which induce in the liver at the translation level have no effect in erythroid tissue. It is assumed that this control at the translation level in the liver is related in some way to microsomal oxidation of foreign substances and to the degradation of haem during these processes. In the

73

liver microsomal oxidative enzymes are present, while their presence was not proved in erythroid tissue. It seems that in erythroid tissue translation regulation of haem synthesis mediated by haem does not exist (*Sassa* and *Granick*, 1970, 1971).

The translation control of ALA synthetase synthesis by iron was suggested in experiments by *Takaku* and *Nakao* (1971). These Japanese workers proved that addition of iron induced an increased incorporation of glycine-^{14}C into haem in bone-marrow cells and in the mitochondrial fraction of bone marrow of patients with iron deficiency. Administration of iron did not influence incorporation in normal bone marrow. At the same time addition of iron did not influence incorporation of ALA-^{14}C into haem of bone marrow cells of patients with iron deficiency anaemia. *Takaku* and *Nakao* assume therefore that iron stimulates the first stage of haem synthesis, ALA synthesis.

Complete inhibition of this induction by iron after addition of puromycin is considered as evidence that the increased rate of haem synthesis after addition of iron depends on protein synthesis. Actinomycin D had no effect on this iron-induced increase in haem synthesis which indicates that the increased incorporation of glycine-^{14}C need not be associated with RNA synthesis. The assumption was made that iron enhances the activity of ALA synthetase by increasing the formation of this enzyme at the translation level.

CHANGES IN ENZYME ACTIVITY

It is generally assumed that haem regulates its own synthesis in erythroid cells by inhibition of ALA synthetase or other enzymes of the synthetic porphyrin chain by end-product inhibition. The first evidence for this concept was provided by experiments of *Lascelles* (1960) who demonstrated that *Rhodopseudomonas spheroides* accumulates porphyrins in the medium during cultivation under conditions of iron deficiency. Addition of small amounts of iron to the suspension reduced porphyrin accumulation to a considerable extent. The possibility was therefore considered that iron facilitates increased synthesis of haem − i.e. the final product of the metabolic chain, and that haem, on the other hand, inhibits by feedback the activity of the first enzyme of the porphyrin chain, ALA synthetase.

Burnham and *Lascelles* (1963) found that in purified cell extract from *Rhodopseudomonas spheroides* haem regulates its own synthesis in two ways: by the repression of ALA synthetase formation, and by the mechanism of inhibition by the endproduct. Inhibition by haem in this system is not competitive but is reversible when heam is diluted. This reversibility of the effect of haem is further evidence that haem acts as a control factor because reversibility is a classical feature of regulatory feedbacks. Haem (ferroprotoporphyrin) is equally effective as haemin (ferriprotoporphyrin). On the other hand, protoporphyrin is much less effective.

74

Granick (1966) did not find any evidence for the inhibition of ALA synthetase by haemin and other metalloporphyrins by the mechanism of inhibition by the end-product. He made his investigations on liver tissue (*Granick*, 1966). Later he demonstrated in collaboration with *Sassa* (*Sassa* and *Granick*, 1970) that addition of haem to isolated mitochondria from liver cells with induced porphyrin synthesis does not influence the activity of ALA synthetase; a certain inhibitory effect of haemin was observed only after addition of unusually high, non-physiological concentrations.

In our laboratory the effect of haemin on ALA synthetase in insoluble particles containing mitochondria prepared from rabbit reticulocytes was investigated. In this system haem in concentrations from 0.1 to 0.4 mM did not exert an inhibitory effect (Table 7; *Neuwirt et al.*, 1969).

Table 7

The effect of various concentrations of haemin on the activity of δ-aminolaevulinic acid synthetase in insoluble particles prepared from rabbit reticulocytes

| Substrate | δ-aminolaevulinic acid product with haemin concentrations of: | | | |
| | 0 | 10^{-4}M | $2 . 10^{-4}$M | $4 . 10^{-4}$M |
	nmoles/mg protein/h			
Citrate	0.729 ± 0.012 (100.0%)	0.892 ± 0.007 (122.3%)	0.987 ± 0.008 (135.5%)	0.803 ± 0.013 (110.1%)
Succinate	0.799 ± 0.018 (100.0%)	0.814 ± 0.011 (101.8%)	1.040 ± 0.148 (130.0%)	1.099 ± 0.059 (137.5%)

(From *Neuwirt et al.*, 1969a. Reproduced with the permission of Springer-Verlag, Heidelberg.)

Bottomley and *Smithee* (1968) studied ALA synthetase in mitochondria of rabbit bone marrow and also in this system they did not find an inhibitory effect of haemin on ALA synthetase in concentrations which varied between 0.01–1 mM haemin.

Welland and *Schwartz* (1966) assessed the activity of ALA synthetase in rabbit reticulocytes with phenylhydrazine anaemia and found inhibition of ALA synthetase after addition of haemin in concentration between 0.01 to 1 mM.

Jones and *Jones* (1970) showed that mitochondrial haem synthetase prepared from rat liver suffers an inhibition of more than 50% by addition of 16 µM protohaem, and ALA synthetase from porphyric mitochondria was inhibited by 10 µM protohaem to an extent of 40%. Inhibition of haem synthetase by protohaem explains, according to these workers, why during porphyria, a condition associated with elevated concentrations of ALA synthetase, porphyrins but not haemins are excreted.

75

According to reports from some laboratories haemin inhibits partly purified ALA synthetase. *Bottomley* and *Smithee* (1969) purified ALA synthetase from rabbit bone marrow. While in isolated mitochondria haemin has no effect, partly purified enzyme is inhibited even at a concentration of 10^{-5} M.

Aoki et al. (1971) purified ALA synthetase from rabbit reticulocytes and increased the activity 4400 times. Haemin in a concentration of 10^{-5} M inhibited the activity of the purified enzyme by 40%. *Aoki et al.* assume that differences in the inhibition by haemin may be due to differences in the degree of ALA synthetase purification.

Irving and *Elliot* (1969) purified ALA synthetase solubilized by sonication and by means of chromatography on Sephadex G-100. The above authors also described an inhibitory effect of haemin.

On the other hand, *Porra et al.* (1973) found that addition of haem does not influence porphyrin production in *Saccharomyces cerevisiae*. They showed that in yeast haem even increased the activity of ALA synthetase and assumed that haem might react allosterically with the enzyme and thus increase its activity.

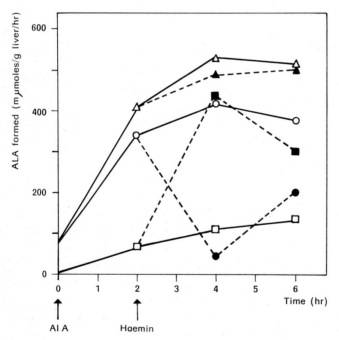

Fig. 28. Effects of haemin on the level of ALA synthetase in the mitochondrial and extramitochondrial fractions. Rats received haemin 2 hours after AIA as indicated by the arrows. —○—, mitochondrial, AIA alone; --●--, mitochondrial, AIA and haemin; ——□——, extramitochondrial, AIA alone; --■--, extramitochondrial, AIA and haemin; ——△——, total, AIA alone; --▲--, total, AIA and haemin. (From *Kurashima et al.*, 1970. Reproduced with the permission of the authors and the Japanese Biochemical Society, Tokyo.)

Several years ago *Hayashi et al.* (1969) made the important observation that in the liver of porphyric rats a high level of soluble ALA synthetase can be detected. *Scholnick et al.* (1969) later confirmed this finding of the Japanese workers in both normal and porphyric rats. These authors proved by detailed experiments that though haemin partly inhibits purified ALA synthetase, its effect can be eliminated by rat and human albumin and cytoplasmatic cell extract. That inhibitory effect of haemin can be prevented by haemin is explained by the fact that albumin and cytoplasmatic proteins combine with haemin and thus reduce its concentration and eliminate its inhibitory effect on ALA synthetase. This finding may partly explain various discrepancies in experiments to demonstrate the inhibitory effect of haem and in particular why haemin does not affect not-purified preparations of ALA synthetase.

ALA synthetase in cytoplasm is probably an enzyme which travels from ribosomes to mitochondria. As some experiments suggested that there exist two ALA synthetases, a mitochondrial and cytoplasmatic one, it will also probably be necessary to re-evaluate all findings pertaining to the regulatory role of haemin and its assumed inhibition of these enzymes (Fig. 28). So far it is not clear how permeable the mitochondrial membrane is for haemin. Haemin may, however, act on ALA synthetase in the cytoplasm, before it enters the mitochondria and this was confirmed by *Scholnick's* experiments (*see also* p. 63). It must be also taken into consideration that both important enzymes of porphyrin metabolism, ALA synthetase and haem synthetase, are located on the inner mitochondrial membrane. The high haem concentration at this site could play an important regulatory role, while haem need not have any detectable effects in isolated systems *in vitro*.

Some workers maintain that haemin can also inhibit the other stages of porphyrin metabolism. *Vavra* (1967) showed that haem can influence an even earlier stage than ALA synthesis. He proved the effect of haemin on succinyl-CoA synthetase. On the other hand, *Calissano et al.* (1966) found that haem has an inhibitory effect on ALA dehydrase from human red cells.

All observations of the inhibitory action of haemin on partly purified ALA synthetase are important. It must, however, be emphasized that haemin even in relatively low concentration has an inhibitory effect on a number of other enzymes such as succinate dehydrogenase, isocitrate dehydrogenase and NADH-cytochrome c reductase (*Silverstein*, 1962). These findings suggest that the action of haem on ALA synthetase need not be specific. Only if the effect of haem on ALA synthetase in intact cells can be demonstrated, will it be possible to speak of specific inhibition of this enzyme by haem and the regulatory role of haemin at this level.

In some laboratories labelled glycine and labelled ALA were used to prove inhibition of ALA synthetase by haem in erythroid cells. *Karibian* and *London* (1965) demonstrated in rabbit reticulocytes significantly inhibited glycine-2-^{14}C utilization for haem synthesis in the presence of haemin. On the other hand, the effect of haem on ALA-4-^{14}C utilization was by no means so marked. This group of workers reported

Table 8

The utilization of glycine-2-^{14}C or δ-amino(4-^{14}C)leavulinate for haem synthesis in the presence of various inhibitors

Exp. No.	Labelled substrate used*	Incorporation (% of control)							
		Conc. . 10^4(M) of haemin				Conc. . 10^3(M) of INH			2 . 10^{-4}M cyclohexamide
		1	2	3	4	1	2	3	
1	Gly			82.1		69.1		34.0	
	ALA			76.0		100.0		77.4	
2	Gly	98.0		75.0			56.7		62.7
	ALA	87.0		69.8			97.9		73.8
3	Gly	88.8	62.4		49.0	40.1			68.8
	ALA	72.1	70.1		50.4	84.4			81.6
4	Gly	75.8	60.6		47.7	42.8			41.1
	ALA	92.9	70.5		53.7	129.0			84.8

Reticulocytes were preincubated with the inhibitors for 15 min before the addition of the label. The inhibitors were present in the mixture during the further 60 min of incubation with the label. The results are expressed as percentages of control values. Each value is based on values from three samples.
*Gly, glycine-2-^{14}C; ALA, δ-amino(4-^{14}C)laevulinate.
(From *Poňka et al.*, 1973. Reproduced with the permission of Elsevier/North-Holland Biomedical Press B.V., Amsterdam.)

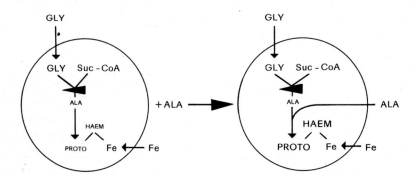

Fig. 29. Schematic representation of the effect of added ALA on the rate of haem formation in intact reticulocytes incubated with a specific inhibitor of ALA synthetase. If haem synthesis is inhibited by some inhibitor before ALA is formed, then the addition of exogenous ALA should restore the inhibition of ^{59}Fe incorporation into haem. This will be correct only if reticulocytes can utilize exogenous ALA for haem synthesis. Table 9 and Fig. 30 provide evidence that exogenous ALA can be utilized for haem synthesis in reticulocytes with inhibited formation of endogenous ALA due to addition of INH. (From *Poňka et al.*, 1973. Reproduced with the permission of the Elsevier/North-Holland Biomedical Press B.V., Amsterdam.)

moreover that during inhibition of globin synthesis in reticulocytes, leading to an increase of the endogenous haem pool in these cells, the incorporation of labelled glycine and labelled ALA into haem follows a similar pattern as after administration of exogenous haemin (*Grayzel et al.*, 1967). These results were interpreted to provide indirect evidence of inhibited ALA formation by haem.

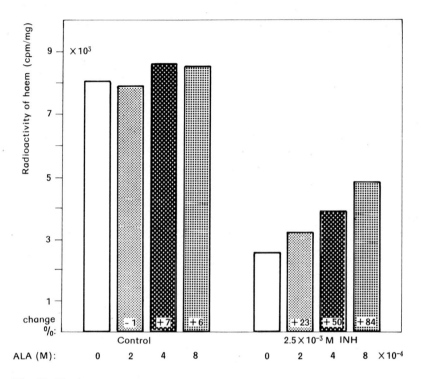

Fig. 30. The incorporation of radioiron into haem of normal or INH treated reticulocytes incubated with various concentrations of exogenous δ-aminolaevulinic acid (ALA). (From *Poňka* and *Neuwirt*, 1971b.)

The results from our laboratory are, however, in a conflict with conclusions presented by London's group. The effects of haemin, INH and cycloheximide on the utilization of glycine-2-^{14}C and ALA-4-^{14}C for haem synthesis were compared. Glycine utilization for haem synthesis is inhibited considerably in the presence of INH, much more than ALA utilization (Table 8). This finding corresponds to the fact that INH is a potent inhibitor of ALA synthetase. If haemin also inhibits this enzyme, the results should be the same as after addition of INH. This, however, was not confirmed. After addition of haemin or cycloheximide* to reticulocytes the

* Cycloheximide treatment elevates the level of uncommitted haem in reticulocytes (*see* p. 137).

utilization of ALA-4-^{14}C for haem synthesis was significantly inhibited. While INH inhibited glycine utilization much more intensely than ALA utilization, in the majority of experiments with haem or cycloheximide the differences in glycine and ALA utilization were less marked (Table 8).

It may be assumed that the specific inhibitor of ALA synthetase will considerably reduce glycine-2-^{14}C utilization and conversely increase ALA-4-^{14}C utilization for haem synthesis. This assumption was confirmed by *Najean et al.* (1964). These authors found during inhibition of ALA synthetase an increased utilization of labelled ALA.

Table 9

The effect of added exogenous ALA on the incorporation of radioiron bound to plasma transferrin into haem of reticulocytes incubated with various inhibitors of haem or globin synthesis

Exp. No.	Group	Concentrations of exogenous ALA (. 10^{-4}M)						
		0	2	2.5	4	5	8	10
1	Control	100.0	99.3		107.2		106.5	
(3)	Haemin (10^{-4}M)	77.5	78.9		77.2		79.1	
	INH (2.5 . 10^{-3}M)	32.2	39.5		48.1		59.2	
2	Control	100.0				90.1		77.3
(2)	Haemin (10^{-4}M)	76.0				68.2		59.2
	*Control	100.0				96.7		112.1
	*Haemin (10^{-4}M)	96.5				87.4		104.0
	*Penicillamine (10^{-3}M)	48.1				74.8		102.6
3	Control	100.0	93.9		92.9		80.6	
(3)	Cycloheximide (2 . 10^{-4}M)	47.5	45.1		45.9		46.5	
4	Control	100.0	107.4		103.1		111.3	
(2)	INH (2 . 10^{-3}M)	35.1	40.0		59.8		74.4	
5	Control	100.0		107.6		124.8		118.5
(3)	Haemin (2 . 10^{-4}M)	83.8		85.8		83.7		82.8
	Cycloheximide (2 . 10^{-4}M)	54.4		46.2		45.0		44.9
6	Control	100.0				112.2		121.3
(3)	Cycloheximide (2 . 10^{-4}M)	41.9				47.3		47.5
	*Control	100.0				122.1		119.9
	*Cycloheximide (2 . 10^{-4}M)	71.3				77.4		84.0

The results are expressed as percentages of appropriate controls, i.e. with no additions. The number of samples incubated in each group are given in parentheses. The time of incubation was in all groups 60 min.
* Haem synthesis was estimated from the incorporation of intracellularly accumulated non-haem radioiron into haem (see p. 28).
(From *Poňka et al.*, 1973. Reproduced with the permission of Elsevier/North-Holland Biomedical Press B.V., Amsterdam.)

Addition of haemin or cycloheximide to the incubation mixture, however, does not lead to these presumed changes. It was therefore concluded that in intact reticulocytes haem does not influence the activity of ALA synthetase (*Poňka et al.*, 1973).

This assumption was also confirmed in subsequent trials. If it is true that haem inhibits ALA synthetase activity in intact reticulocytes, then addition of exogeneous ALA to reticulocytes incubated with haemin or cycloheximide should re-establish the normal rate of haem synthesis (Fig. 29). The results of our experiments revealed that addition of exogenous ALA to the incubation mixture almost completely restores haem synthesis in reticulocytes incubated with an inhibitor of ALA synthetase (INH or penicillamine) (Fig. 30). On the other hand, addition of exogenous ALA is not able to restore haem synthesis in reticulocytes incubated with haemin and in reticulocytes with a raised haem level after cycloheximide (Table 9, Fig. 31). Thus in all these experiments no evidence of the inhibitory effect of haem on ALA synthetase in intact erythroid cells was found.

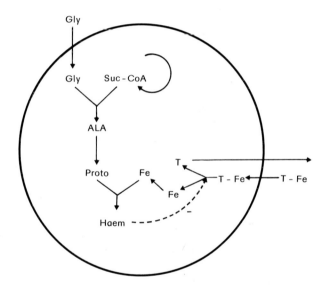

Fig. 31. The role of haem in the intracellular metabolism of iron. The inhibitory effect of haem on the release of iron from transferrin need not be a direct one, but haem can interfere with a metabolic step required for the release of iron (*see* p. 45). Gly − glycine; Suc-CoA − succinyl-coenzyme A; ALA − δ-aminolaevulinic acid; Proto − protoporphyrin IX; T = transferrin; T-Fe = iron-transferrin complex. (From *Poňka et al.*, 1974. Reproduced with the permission of S. Karger AG, Basle.)

In the chapter on iron uptake by erythroid cells evidence was submitted that exogenous and endogenous haems limit the process of iron release from transferrin in reticulocytes and thus control iron uptake. The problem whether this effect of haem on iron uptake inhibits haem synthesis in the cell will be discussed in the following section. The concept of feed-back regulation of haem synthesis at the level of iron uptake requires the evidence that: (1) the rate of iron uptake limits the rate of haem synthesis in reticulocytes, and (2) haem does not decrease the utilization of intracellular non-haem iron for haem synthesis.

The idea that haem synthesis is controlled by iron uptake was first submitted by *Klein* (1961). Some of our results support this idea and suggest that the iron supply to the site of haem synthesis may be the limiting factor which controls the rate of haem synthesis. Evidence was provided that lack of plasma iron reduces the utilization of labelled glycine for haem synthesis (*Poňka* and *Neuwirt*, 1970). On the other hand, it was found (*see* p. 32) that reticulocytes with an artificially raised non-haem iron pool incorporate more glycine-2-^{14}C into haem than normal reticulocytes.

Addition of exogenous ALA to reticulocytes *in vitro* does not increase ^{59}Fe incorporation into haem (*Poňka, Neuwirt* and *Borová*, 1973). Similarly, in patients with erythropoietic porphyria the normal rate of haem synthesis is maintained under conditions of great porphyrin overproduction. As it can be hardly assumed that haem synthetase limits the rate of haem production (*see* p. 68), both examples mentioned above suggest that the rate of haem synthesis is controlled by the capacity of the cell to take up iron and/or deliver it to the site of haem synthesis in mitochondria.

To demonstrate the feedback regulation of haem synthesis by haem at the level of iron uptake by the cell another experimental approach was selected. The effect of haem on reticulocytes with an artificially raised precursor non-haem iron pool was tested (*see* p. 28). In these reticulocytes the actual rate of haem synthesis can be investigated while all factors which affect the transport of iron from the incubation medium into the cell interior are eliminated. Table 10 shows that haem inhibits ^{59}Fe incorporation from transferrin into haem while in the same concentration it has no effect on incorporation of radioiron into haem from the intracellular non-haem iron pool. These results indicate that inhibition of iron uptake by haem causes inhibition of haem synthesis.

Furthermore it was found that haemin has only a mild inhibitory effect on the incorporation of glycine-2-^{14}C into haem of reticulocytes with an artificially increased non-haem iron pool (*see* Table 10). It is possible that the slight inhibition of labelled glycine utilization in these reticulocytes is not a sign of reduced haem synthesis but is more likely due to interference of haem with glycine uptake by reticulocytes (*see* Fig. 21).

82

Table 10

The effect of haemin on glycine-2-^{14}C incorporation into haem of reticulocytes with normal or elevated non-haem iron and on the utilization of ^{59}Fe bound to transferrin or present in the non-haem iron pool

Concentration of haemin	Incorporation into haem			
	Glycine-2-^{14}C into:		^{59}Fe from:	
	Normal cells	Cells preincubated	Transferrin	Intracellular non-haem pool
1 . 10^{-4}M	67.0 (4)	93.7 (4)	66.6 (4)	93.5 (4)
2 . 10^{-4}M	38.3 (2)	63.0 (2)	44.6 (4)	100.7 (4)

1/6 — 1/4 of rabbit plasma with or without iron were added to the incubation mixture. The number of experiments are given in parentheses. Values are expressed as the average of percentages of the control group.
(From *Poňka* and *Neuwirt*, 1970. Reproduced with the permission of Blackwell Scientific Publications Ltd., Oxford.)

Table 11

Comparison of the effects of exo- and endogenous haem and INH on various metabolic parameters in reticulocytes incubated *in vitro*

Addition	Iron uptake	Transferrin uptake	Iron release	HCO₃ release	Iron incorp. into mitochondria	Utilization for haem synthesis of		
						Transferrin-bound iron	Intracellular non-haem iron	Exogenous ALA
Haemin	↓	↑	↓	↓	↓	↓ ¹)	normal	↓
Cyclo-heximide (↑ Endo. haem)	↓	normal or ↑	↓	↓	?	↓ ¹)	normal or slightly ↓	↓
INH	↑	normal or ↓	↑	↑	↑	↓ ²)	↓	not inhibited, in some cases ↑

¹) This inhibition cannot be eliminated by exogenous ALA
²) This inhibition can be eliminated by exogenous ALA

Subsequent experiments also revealed that endogenous intracellular haem which accumulates during incubation of reticulocytes with cycloheximide does not significantly reduce the utilization of intracellular non-haem radioiron for haem synthesis (*Neuwirt et al.*, 1969; *Poňka* and *Neuwirt*, 1971).

Differences in the action of haem (exogenous and endogenous) and of INH must be again emphasized. Table 11 shows clearly that INH which is a well-defined inhibitor of ALA synthetase influences various parameters in a quite different way than haem.

All results so far obtained correspond to the concept that in intact reticulocytes under physiological conditions haem synthesis is controlled by haem, in the sense that haem controls the iron uptake by the cell (Fig. 31). Our results suggest on the contrary that serious doubts may be raised as regards the hitherto generally accepted concept of the feedback inhibition of ALA synthetase by haem. It is unlikely that under physiological conditions in intact erythroid cells haem synthesis is controlled by the end-product inhibition of ALA synthetase.

In this connection it must be mentioned that haem in relatively low concentrations also inhibits glycine transport into reticulocytes (*see* p. 51). It seems, however, that haem synthesis is not affected by this effect of haem on glycine transport (*Neuwirt* and *Poňka*, 1972).

METABOLIC AND EXTERNAL FACTORS

All functions of haem are closely related to oxidation processes and it may thus be assumed that cellular oxidation may influence the metabolic regulation of haem and porphyrin synthesis. So far, however, no regulatory mechanism has been described which could confirm the association of porphyrin and haem synthesis with biological oxidation processes. There is only some indirect evidence. *Falk et al.* (1959) showed that in avian red cells incubated *in vitro* the reduction of oxygen tension to a certain level increases porphyrin and haem synthesis.

One of the important regulatory factors of haem synthesis is the availability of bivalent Fe^{2+} for haem synthetase. This availability of bivalent iron may be influenced by the oxygen concentration near mitochondria and by electron transport at the terminal chain.

The availability of glycine, succinate or succinyl-CoA could also potentially limit haem synthesis. *Kappas et al.* (1968), however, conclude that control at this site is unlikely because: a) probably less than 1% succinyl-CoA formed in cells is used for haem synthesis and therefore changes in the production of succinyl-CoA would not be a very effective control mechanism. b) Succinate is formed in Krebs cycle and every metabolic change would be reflected in haem synthesis and this too does not suggest control by this route. c) It is unlikely that haem synthesis is controlled by regulation of glycine uptake by cells. Our own results revealed that regulation of the glycine supply to erythroid cells is not of major importance for the regulation of haem synthesis. A certain role could be played by regulation of glycine transport across the mitochondrial membrane.

The presence of SH substances is necessary for the activity of some enzymes of porphyrin metabolism. Under pathological conditions, e.g. in lead intoxication, inhibition of SH enzymes has an adverse effect on porphyrin synthesis.

The availability of pyridoxal phosphate and some other factors can also play a part in the control of haem synthesis. It seems, however, that under normal conditions pyridoxal phosphate is available in sufficient amounts.

Finally the last possible regulatory mechanism could be the breakdown of ALA by some other metabolic pathway (*Shemin* and *Russell*, 1953). 90% of ALA is used under normal conditions for haem synthesis. So far there is no evidence that this ratio is reduced in certain conditions and that this influences haem synthesis.

In cells there is normally a very low porphobilinogen level and its amount increases only during porphyria. *Frydman et al.* (1973) provided evidence that during increased ALA synthetase activity and enhanced porphobilinogen production the latter may be transformed by porphobilinogen oxygenase to pyrrolinone derivatives which are not converted further to porphyrins. Porphobilinogen oxygenase was isolated from rat liver where it is present in microsomes in the inhibited form. Some substances, e.g. phenobarbital, reduce the amount of inhibitor of this enzyme and porphobilinogen is then converted to pyrrolinone substances. The physiological concentration of porphobilinogen for haem synthesis is very important and therefore the oxidation of porphobilinogen to non-porphyrin substances during induced porphyrin synthesis may act as an important regulating factor.

HAEM CATABOLISM

In recent years the exact mechanism of haem conversion from haemoglobin and other haem proteins to bilirubin was revealed. This conversion takes place in a number of tissues. For haem oxidation the presence of two NADPH-dependent enzymes is necessary. The first of these is haem oxygenase which is present in the membranes of the endoplasmatic reticulum; it is insoluble and can be induced by substrate. This protein binds haem stereospecifically and forms a complex with it which can use molecular oxygen, NADPH and the microsomal electron transport system to be converted into α-hydroxyhaem. The unstable α-hydroxyhaem reacts spontaneously with molecular oxygen and loses CO and then Fe^{3+} by hydrolysis. The IX-α-biliverdin which is formed is reduced to bilirubin IX-α by the soluble enzyme biliverdin reductase (*Schmid* and *McDonaugh*, 1975).

So far it has not been proved that haem is broken down by this mechanism in erythroid cells. Haem from haemoglobin in erythroid cells is catabolized by this mechanism by reticuloendothelial cells. If it were possible to demonstrate that in erythroid cell enzymes are present which break down haem we should have to change some of our ideas on the regulation of haem synthesis. These ideas are based on the assumption that haem synthesis is regulated by a pool of "uncommitted" (free?) haem, the level of which is determined by the anabolic pathway only.

4. GLOBIN SYNTHESIS

GLOBIN BIOSYNTHESIS

GENERAL INTRODUCTION

Proteins are synthesized by a very similar mɔchanism in all living systems. There are, ho vever, two different protein producing systems: prokaryotes (e.g. bacteria) and eukaryotes; the latter include cells of higher organisms and also erythroid cells which synthesize globin. These two protein synthesizing systems differ mainly with regard to structural properties of their ribosomes and their sensitivity to antibiotics.

It is generally known that in the nucleotide sequence of the deoxyribonucleic acid (DNA) molecule (gene) information for protein formation (thus also for globin) is present. Genes are located on the chromosome inside the cell nucleus. DNA is a double stranded polymer in which four different deoxyribonucleotides (dC, dA, dG, dT) are arranged in a linear array or nucleotide sequence (*Watson*, 1970). Genetic information contained in DNA is transmitted by the process of transcription into the nucleotide sequence of messenger ribonucleic acid (mRNA) which contains four different ribonucleotides (C, A, G, U). mRNA is formed by transcription of the gene according to rules of complementarity, i.e. each deoxyribonucleotide of DNA is represented by its complementary ribonucleotide in the messenger RNA (dC gives G, dA gives U, dG gives C and dT gives A). Individual nucleotides (in both DNA and RNA) are united by means of a phosphate diester linkage between carbon atom 3 of one sugar molecule and a terminal carbon (5) of the next. This means that at one end of the polynucleotide chain there is a free hydroxyl group on the fifth carbon atom of the sugar and at the other end there is a free 3'-group. This asymmetry of the molecule is important because it enables the cells to differentiate correctly between the "beginning" and "end" of the polynucleotide sequence in the process of decoding: DNA transcription starts from the 3'-end, while mRNA is translated in the 5' to 3' direction.

Messenger RNA migrates outside the nucleus into the cytoplasm where, in association with ribosomal RNA, it acts as a template to direct the synthesis of the specific protein (globin). The sequence of purine and pyrimidine bases on the mRNA strand (determined by the information transcribed from the nuclear DNA) is decisive for the primary structure, i.e. the sequence of amino acids in the protein. This process of decoding of information contained in the mRNA molecule is called translation. The principle of translation of information from the mRNA molecule into the molecule of the specific protein (e.g. globin) is that each successive sequence of three nucleotides (triplets, codons) in the mRNA codes for one amino acid. Sixty one

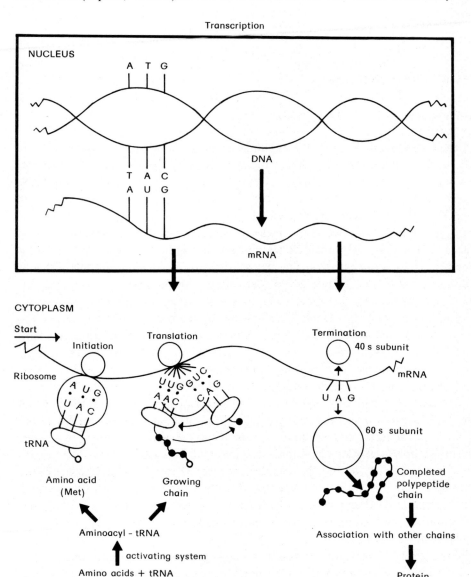

Fig. 32. General outline of protein synthesis. Details of the various reactions are discussed in subsequent text. (From *Benz* and *Forget*, 1974. Reproduced with the permission of the authors and W. B. Saunders Publishing Co., Philadelphia.)

88

of 64 possible triplets code for 20 amino acids required in the synthesis of proteins which means that each amino acid can be represented by more than one triplet; each codon specifies, however, only one amino acid.

Amino acids interact with codons indirectly in association with the molecule of transfer RNA (tRNA). For each codon there is a specific tRNA which recognizes the codon because it contains the complementary nucleotide sequence (anti-codon). The interaction of mRNA and amino acyl-tRNA is mediated by the ribosome. The polypeptide chain grows on the ribosome by successive addition of individual amino acids, while at the same time this multimacromolecular complex moves along mRNA. Polypeptide synthesis begins from the amino-terminal amino acid and proceeds in the direction towards the carboxy-terminal amino acid. In the subsequent paragraphs this general pattern of protein synthesis (Fig. 32) which also applies to globin synthesis will be discussed in more detail.

ROLE OF RIBONUCLEIC ACIDS IN GLOBIN SYNTHESIS

In protein synthesis three different types of ribonucleic acids (RNA) which differ in structural, metabolic and functional properties participate. Ribosomal RNA (rRNA) is quantitatively most important and is present in minute cytoplasmatic particles, ribosomes. rRNAs are discussed in more detail in the chapter dealing with ribosomes (p. 109). The next most abundant type is the "soluble", "transfer" or "acceptor" RNA (tRNA) which carries each amino acid to the proper site during polypeptide synthesis. "Messenger" RNA accounts for less than 5% of the total RNA in the cell. It is, however, a very important fraction because it is a quite specific factor, determining protein structure.

Messenger RNA

The term messenger RNA (mRNA) was introduced into molecular biology by *Jacob* and *Monod* (1961). These workers elaborated a theory of genetic mechanisms, based on experimental results assembled by various workers, which control protein synthesis. The RNA fraction with messenger properties was originally demonstrated in bacteria (*Brenner et al.*, 1961) but later a great deal of evidence was collected that a similar RNA fraction should also be present in mammalian cells.

In attempts to isolate mRNA from mammalian sources the main attention of workers was focused on the isolation of mRNA for globin from reticulocytes. This cell was selected because reticulocytes synthesize practically only haemoglobin (*Kruh* and *Borsook*, 1956; *Dintzis*, 1961). Haemoglobin synthesis in reticulocytes depends on mRNA formed before this cellular stage, because reticulocytes do not synthesize any new mRNA (*Marks et al.*, 1962) the synthesis of which is completed before the stage of the orthochromic normoblast (*DeBellis et al.*, 1964). These facts suggest that the reticulocyte should serve as a very favourable system for the isolation of mRNA: nature selected a longliving "messenger" for a known protein which probably is not contamined by other "messengers". Another great advantage is the easy separation of reticulocytes. As a matter of fact the first eukaryotic messenger ribonucleic acid which was isolated and identified was globin mRNA from reticulocytes.

In the literature after 1963 a large number of papers on mRNA for globin was published and we shall mention only the most important data concerning globin mRNA.

Isolation and identification of globin mRNA

In search on globin mRNA workers used two basically different approaches. One group of workers tried to develop suitable systems for the detection of globin mRNA, while others tried to isolate globin mRNA from reticulocytes, with regard to its expected properties. The successive development of these two branches of research and advances in the isolation (*Huez et al.*, 1967; *Chantrenne et al.*, 1967), characterisation (*Labrie*, 1969) and translation of mRNA in different systems (*Lockard* and *Lingrel*, 1969; 1971; *Mathews et al.*, 1971; *Gurdon et al.*, 1971) greatly contributed towards the elucidation of one of the most important problems of protein and haemoglobin synthesis.

Chantrenne, Burny and *Marbaix* in 1967 summarized their attempts to isolate globin mRNA. Their preparation had many properties which suggested "messenger RNA": (1) it accounted for cca 3% of the total RNA, (2) its turnover in bone marrow cells was greater than the turnover of ribosomal RNA, (3) it was preferentially broken down after the action of pancreatic ribonuclease on ribosomes, (4) it was released from polyribosomes when Mg^{2+} ions were taken up by means of EDTA, (5) it sedimented as a homogeneous substance with a sedimentation constant (9 s), which corresponded roughly to the expected "messenger" for individual haemoglobin chains.

In other laboratories it proved possible to develop many cell-free systems which synthesized proteins (*Schaeffer et al.*, 1964; *Drach* and *Lingrel*, 1964; 1966a, 1966b; *Brawerman et al.*, 1965; *Kruh et al.*, 1964). Addition of various fractions of reticulocyte RNA to cell-free systems stimulated the amino acid incorporation into proteins. It must be, however, emphasized that many properties of some effective RNA fractions did not correspond to the anticipated properties of mRNA (*Drach* and *Lingel*, 1966b). Stimulation of amino acid incorporation into proteins cannot be considered evidence of enhanced haemoglobin synthesis and moreover added reticulocyte RNA may protect endogenous mRNA of a given cell-free system against inactivation. From this ensued that one of the unequivocal criteria for the detection of mRNA is stimulation of haemoglobin synthesis (not only amino acid incorporation) in a system which contains no mRNA for the appropriate globin.

The first convincing evidence that the RNA fraction stimulated mRNA-dependent globin synthesis in a heterologous system was presented by *Lockard* and *Lingrel* (1969). These workers demonstrated that 9 s RNA isolated from polysomes of mouse reticulocytes controlled the formation of β-chains of mouse haemoglobin in a cell-free system of rabbit reticulocytes. Newly synthesized β-chains which were formed in the presence of mouse 9 s mRNA were identical with β-chains of mouse globin as was demonstrated conclusively by electrophoresis of tryptic digest of the formed product (*Lockard* and *Lingrel*, 1971). In this system α-chains of mouse globin are also synthesized.

More recently many other workers have confirmed these results. Translation of exogenous mRNA for haemoglobin was also achieved in various other cell-free systems (*Mathews et al.*, 1971; *Efron* and *Marcus*, 1973), as will be discussed later. Moreover, an excellent cellular system for testing translation of globin mRNA was developed (*Lane, Marbaix* and *Gurdon*, 1971; *Moar et al.*, 1971).

Methods used for the isolation of globin mRNA

Globin mRNA is prepared most frequently from polyribosomes which are obtained from a reticulocyte lysate by sedimentation through sucrose gradients. By the action of sodium dodecyl sulphate (SDS) on polyribosomes globin mRNA can be released (*Marbaix* and *Burny*, 1964). SDS is an anionic detergent, a nuclease inhibitor, and releases nucleic acids from their association with protein or lipoprotein structures. Further separation of RNA SDS-protein complexes is achieved by zonal centrifugation in a sucrose gradient. This procedure is suitable for the isolation of globin mRNA which has a sedimentation constant of 9 s and therefore is readily separated from ribosomal RNA (Fig. 33).

Alternatively by the action of EDTA on polyribosomes globin mRNA is released in the form of a ribonucleoprotein complex with a sedimentation constant of 15 s (*Chantrenne et al.*, 1967; *Labrie*, 1969). The stability of ribosomes depends among others on the Mg^{2+} ion concentration. EDTA reduces their concentration below a critical level and dissociates ribosomes into two ribosomal sub-units, whereby the ribonucleoprotein complex containing mRNA is released. The released complex can be separated from ribosomal sub-units and transfer RNA by centrifugation on a sucrose gradient. This ribonucleoprotein complex of mRNA was well characterized (*Lebleu et al.*, 1971) and it was shown that it controls the synthesis of globin chains *in vitro* as effectively as free 9 s globin mRNA (*Ernst* and *Arnstein*, 1975).

The stability of two ribosomal sub-units in the active ribosome of polyribosomes depends to a considerable extent on the presence of the nascent polypeptide chain. If the nascent polypeptide chains are released by puromycin in the presence of a high ionic strength, dissociation into ribosomal sub-units takes place and messenger RNA is released in the form of ribonucleoprotein. In the case of mRNA for rabbit globin a ribonucleoprotein with a sedimentation coefficient of 20 s was obtained during the action of a low ionic strength, or that of 11.3 s at the presence of a high ionic strength (*Blobel*, 1971, 1972).

mRNA can also be isolated by extraction with phenol (*Georgiev*, 1962), or by centrifugation over a layer of caesium chloride (*Glišin et al.*, 1974). mRNA is then usually purified by affinity chromatography on poly(U)-Sepharose. Both these methods can be used for the isolation of mRNA from the whole cell homogenate.

Recently methods have become very popular which make use of the finding that mRNAs are the only cytoplasmatic type of RNA which contain a poly(A) segment

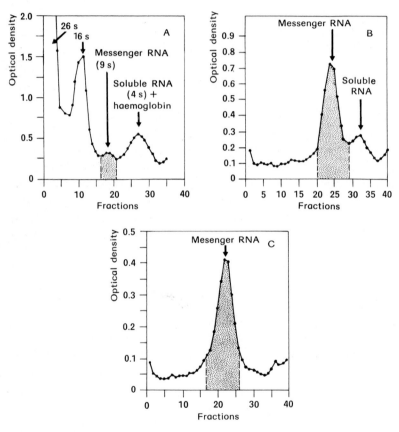

Fig. 33. Purification of mRNA by three successive sucrose gradient centrifugations: (A) first centrifugation, (B) second centrifugation, (C) third centrifugation. Centrifugations were performed in linear 8−20% sucrose gradients equilibrated in 5 mM Tris-HCl, pH 7,4 (40 hours at 24,000 rpm (60,000 × g) in the Spinco rotor SW 25.1 at 4°). After each centrifugation, the material corresponding to the hatched area was dialyzed and lyophilized. It was then submitted to the next centrifugation. (From *Marbaix et al.*, 1966. Reproduced with the permission of the authors and Elsevier/North-Holland Biomedical Press B. V., Amsterdam.)

(see below). The RNA mixture can be adsorbed either on oligo(dT) bound to cellulose (*Aviv* and *Leder*, 1972) or poly(U) bound to glass fibre filters, to cellulose or covalently bound to Sepharose (*Sheldon et al.*, 1972; *Lindberg* and *Persson*, 1972) under conditions of high ionic strength, i.e. under conditions promoting the formation of hydrogen bonds between complementary bases (hybridization). Bound messenger RNA is then released by elution at low ionic strenght or by a combination of low ionic strength and gradual increase of temperature to achieve higher yields (*Morrison et al.*, 1972).

For isolation of mRNA adsorption on nitrocellulose membrane filters in the presence of 0.5 M KCl can also be used. Material containing poly(A) segment shorter than 50 nucleotides, however, passes without being retained (*Gorski et al.*, 1974).

Globin mRNA isolated by these methods is a mixture of messenger ribonucleic acids for α- and β-chains of haemoglobin. The separation of these two mRNA species can be achieved after treatment of rabbit reticulocytes with O-methyl-threonine. O-methyl-threonine is an isoleucine analogue (*Rabinovitz et al.*, 1969) (*see also* p. 111) which blocks aminoacylation of isoleucine tRNA. In certain species of rabbits isoleucine is near the NH_2-end of the 141 amino acid α-chain (in positions 10, 17 and 55) and at the COOH-end of the 146 amino acid β-chain in position 112. As protein synthesis begins with the amino-terminal amino acid and proceeds toward the carboxy-terminal amino acid, inhibition of the movement of ribosomes on the messenger RNA occurs near the initiation end of mRNA for the α-chain and conversely at the 3'-end of mRNA for the β-chain. This leads to the formation of disomes and trisomes on the α-chain mRNA, while the β-chain mRNA is overburdened and contains roughly 12 ribosomes (Fig. 34, *Kazazian* and *Freedman*, 1968). Both classes of polyribosomes can be separated by centrifugation and then messenger RNA for α- and β-globin chains can be isolated. The mRNA obtained is, however, not quite pure and contains ca 20% mRNA for the second globin chain (*Temple* and *Housman*, 1972).

Relatively pure mRNA for the α-chain of globin can be isolated from the post-ribosomal supernatant of rabbit reticulocyte lysate. Rabbit reticulocytes contain

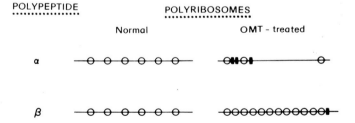

Fig. 34. The change in α- and β-chain polyribosomes in reticulocytes incubared with L-O-methyl-threonine (OMT) is shown on the right. (From *Kazazian* and *Freedman*, 1968. Reproduced with the permission of the authors and the American Society of Biological Chemists, Inc., Bethesda.)

globin mRNA which is not linked to ribosomes and is in a form of ribonucleoprotein with a sedimentation constant of ca 20 s. This "supernatant" globin mRNA mainly controls synthesis of the α-chain, the β-chain accounts for 0–30% of the total amount of synthesized globin (*Jacobs-Lorena* and *Baglioni*, 1972; *Bonanou-Tzedaki et al.*, 1972; *Gianni et al.*, 1972, *Olsen et al.*, 1972; *Sherman et al.*, 1974). Recently *Huez et al.* (1976) reported that in mammalian reticulocytes free mRNA represents mainly the last stage of the message life.

Recently for the separation of polyribosomes synthesizing α- and β-chains of rabbit haemoglobin an immunochemical method was used (*Boyer et al.*, 1974). The use of chain specific antibodies renders specific precipitation of polyribosomes synthesizing α- or β-chains of rabbit haemoglobin possible.

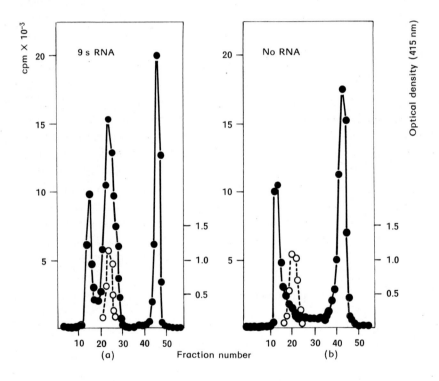

Fig. 35. The Sephadex G-100 elution profiles obtained from homogenates of oocytes injected with haemin and 9 s RNA and of controls injected with haemin but no RNA. Rabbit haemoglobin was added as a marker. Open circles (——○——○——) refer to optical density at 415 mm and closed circles (——●—●—●——) refer to counts/min. Details of the experimental technique may be found in the original paper. (From *Lane et al.*, 1971b. Reproduced with the permission of the authors and Academic Press, Inc., London.)

94

Detection of messenger RNA for globin

For the detection of globin messenger RNA either the ability of isolated mRNA to control the formation of globin in a cellular system (oocytes) or in various cell-free systems, or methods of molecular hybridization are used.

Cellular system — frog oocytes. *Gurdon et al.* developed an excellent system for testing translation of mRNA (*Lane et al.*, 1971, *Moar et al.*, 1971). These workers demonstrated that oocytes of the frog *Xenopus laevis* injected with rabbit globin mRNA (and haemin) synthesize rabbit haemoglobin. Fig. 35 shows the synthesis of the new component in oocytes into which 9 s globin RNA isolated from rabbit reticulocytes was injected. By means of gel filtration, chromatography on carboxymethyl cellulose and electrophoresis on acrylamide gel evidence was provided that the product formed is actually haemoglobin.

After injection of globin mRNA into oocytes haemoglobin is synthesized (*Lane et al.*, 1971; *Moar et al.*, 1971; *Gurdon et al.*, 1971; *Marbaix* and *Gurdon*, 1972; *Marbaix* and *Lane*, 1972) for many hours to days (*Gurdon et al.*, 1973). Translation of globin messenger RNA takes place in oocytes (at 19°C) four times more slowly than in rabbit reticulocytes (at 37°C) and its addition to the oocyte does not influence the rate of endogenous protein synthesis in oocytes (*Moar et al.*, 1971; *Gurdon*, 1973). The advantages of frog oocytes, compared to cell-free systems, are fewer artefacts and the highly efficient translation for a much longer period than the life span of rabbit reticulocytes. The injected globin mRNA in oocytes is very stable (*Gurdon et al.*, 1973, 1974) and for its translation initiating factors from rabbit reticulocytes are not needed (*Marbaix and Gurdon*, 1972).

Cell-free systems. For translation of isolated globin mRNA preincubated postmitochondrial supernatants of various eukaryotic cells are frequently used, e.g. ascitic mouse cells (*Aviv et al.*, 1971; *Aviv* and *Leder*, 1972; *Metafora et al.*, 1972; *Mathews et al.*, 1970; 1971; 1972; *Mathews*, 1972; *Housman et al.*, 1971), rat and mouse liver cells (*Sampson et al.*, 1972a; 1972b) and wheat embryos (*Efron* and *Marcus*, 1973; *Roberts* and *Paterson*, 1973). By preincubation with the energy source and amino acids the rate of endogenous protein synthesis is reduced and ribosomal sub-units are released which render translation of added globin mRNA possible.

The cell-free system from mouse ascitic cells is obviously deficient in many components because e.g. after addition of transfer RNA (*Metafora et al.*, 1972) and initiating factors from rabbit reticulocytes (*Metafora et al.*, 1972; *Mathews et al.*, 1972; *Lebleu et al.*, 1972; *Knöchel et al.*, 1973) the amount of synthesized globin increases.

Efron and *Marcus* in 1973 were the first to describe the translation of globin mRNA in a cell-free system from wheat embryos. Purified globin mRNA stimulated the incorporation of labelled leucine into proteins about 20 times and the synthesized product was identified as rabbit globin. The advantage of the cell-free system from wheat embryos is the low endogenous protein synthesis because wheat embryos contain only ribosomes without endogenous messenger RNA. The system synthesizes α- and β-chains of rabbit globin at a ratio of 1 : 1.

Synthesis of rabbit globin after addition of globin mRNA was also demonstrated in the postmitochondrial supernatant of the brain of chicken embryos (*Hendrick et al.*, 1974a; 1974b). Whole chains of rabbit globin were synthesized without any special requirement of initiating factors from reticulocytes.

In addition to these postmitochondrial supernatants (which contain polyribosomes) for the translation of globin mRNA postmicrosomal (i.e. post-polyribosomal) supernatant was used (*Burke et al.*, 1973). *Burke et al.* prepared this postmicrosomal supernatant (PMS) under such conditions that it contained native ribosomal subunits which are naturally present in cells (*see* p. 111). In our laboratory *Borová et al.* (1976) were able to increase the effectiveness of this system by addition of a pH 5.1 precipitate of PMS (Fig. 36). At pH 5 all ribonucleoprotein particles (in this case

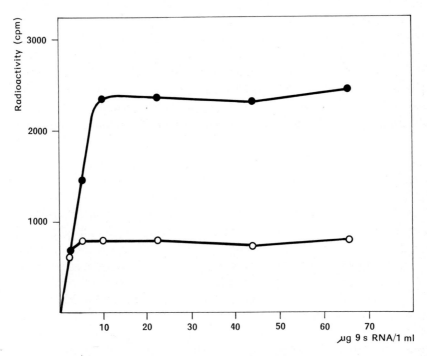

Fig. 36. The saturation of cell-free system with globin mRNA isolated from rabbit reticulocytes. The details concerning composition of the cell-free system, preparation of post-microsomal supernatant (PMS) and enriched PMS may be found in the original paper (*Borová et al.*, 1976). The cell-free system was incubated with leucine-^{14}C and with various amounts of globin mRNA for 20 min at 30°C. Thereafter, the samples (0.1 ml) were withdrawn and the radioactivity incorporated into proteins was determined. ○——○, PMS; ●——●, enriched PMS.

96

native ribosomal sub-units, pH 5 enzymes and transfer RNA) precipitate (*Arnstein et al.*, 1965). PMS from rat liver contains all factors required for translation of rabbit globin RNA (*Burke et al.*, 1973). Fig. 37 provides convincing evidence that in this cell-free system α- and β-chains of rabbit globin are synthesized after addition of rabbit reticulocyte 9 s mRNA. The other RNAs prepared from rabbit reticulocytes do not enhance protein synthesis in this system (*Borová et al.*, 1976; *Fuchs et al.*, 1976).

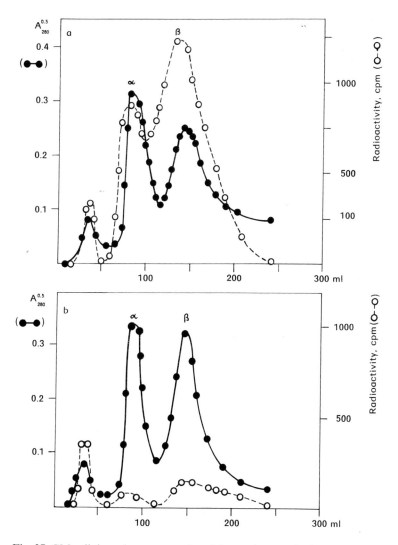

Fig. 37. CM-cellulose chromatography of the product synthesized in the cell-free system (*Borová et al.*, 1976). a, globin mRNA (10 μg per ml of the cell-free system). b, without globin mRNA.

97

In recent years for the detection of template activity of globin mRNA various cell-free systems have been used where individual components were prepared from different sources (e.g. *Heywood*, 1970; *Gilbert* and *Anderson*, 1970; *Prichard et al.*, 1971; *Waldman* and *Goldstein*, 1973; *Schapira et al.*, 1973; *Vaquero et al.*, 1973; *Schreier* and *Staehelin et al.*, 1973a,b,c). For example according to *Schreier* and *Staehelin* a frequently used cell-free system contains ribosomal sub-units from mouse liver, pH 5 enzymes from rat liver (a source of transfer RNA and all factors needed for polypeptide synthesis *in vitro; Falvey* and *Staehelin*, 1970) and initiation factors from rabbit reticulocytes.

The methods used for the preparation of ribosomal sub-units are briefly described elsewhere (p. 111). In this connection it is worth mentioning that *Crystal et al.* (1972) used rabbit reticulocyte ribosomes containing mRNA fragments in their cell-free system. Such ribosomes were prepared after short-term treatment with ribonuclease.

The disadvantage of cell-free systems containing individual isolated or purified components is that many purified constituents (particularly initiation factors) are not sufficiently stable and easily lose their activity during isolation and storage. These systems formed by isolated components of the proteosynthetic apparatus are particularly suited for investigation of basic mechanisms of protein synthesis. On the other hand, for detection of the biological activity of isolated globin mRNA it seems better to use non-purified cell-free systems which are easily prepared and with which a relatively high efficiency of translation of exogenous globin mRNA can be achieved.

In conjunction with translation of globin mRNA in cell-free systems it is appropriate to mention the mode of identification of the product of protein synthesis, haemoglobin. For orientational and rapid testing of globin synthesis in a cell-free system it is sufficient to assess the incorporation of labelled amino acids into total proteins in the presence or absence of globin mRNA.

The product, radioactive globin, is identified usually after addition of haemoglobin as a carrier either unlabelled or labelled by another isotope on the same amino acid. By precipitation with acid acetone globin is prepared which is further analyzed by chromatography on a CM cellulose column (*Dintzis*, 1961; *Clegg et al.*, 1965) or electrophoretically. The radioactivity of the labelled amino acid, incorporated into the product, must be found in the isolated globin chains. The most accurate evidence of *de novo* globin synthesis controlled by added messenger RNA is the appearance of radioactivity in peptides of globin after their breakdown by a proteolytic enzyme (*Schapira et al.*, 1968b). It is an advantage to use double labelling (^{3}H and ^{14}C) and the finding of both isotopes (the carrier and the product) in the same peptides is convincing evidence of the identity of the product.

Investigations of translation of globin mRNA in different cell-free systems and in oocytes revealed that under different conditions the ratio between the formation of α- and β-globin chains differs. Although it seems that the rabbit reticulocyte contains relatively more globin mRNA for the α-chain than for the β-chain (*Lodish*,

1971; *Lodish* and *Nathan*, 1972), in some cell-free systems fewer α- than β-chains of globin are synthesized after addition of total reticulocyte mRNA. In cell-free systems a predominance of β- over α-chain synthesis was observed when the concentration of globin mRNA was high (*Hall* and *Arnstein*, 1973; *McKeehan*, 1974; *Anderson*, 1974; *Ernst* and *Arnstein*, 1975), when there was a quantitative predominance of 60s sub-units over 40s sub-units of ribosomes (*McKeehan*, 1974) and during deficiency of transfer RNA (*Gilbert* and *Anderson*, 1970). Also the concentration of potassium and magnesium ions and the concentration of initiation factors has a great impact on the ratio of α- and β-globin chain synthesis. Predominance of the synthesis of β- over α-chains of rabbit globin is also observed in oocytes at a low haemin concentration (*Giglioni et al.*, 1973; *Lingrel* and *Woodland*, 1974; *Lane et al.*, 1974). These findings are more or less of methodical importance but probably are not relevant for the physiological regulation of globin chain synthesis.

Molecular hybridization. DNA-RNA hybridization is another method which is widely used in recent years for the detection of globin mRNA. Till recently it was not possible to obtain an eukaryotic DNA complementary to individual mRNAs and thus these methods could not be used in eukaryotic systems. However, when it was demonstrated that RNA-dependent DNA polymerase ("reverse transcriptase") synthesizes a copy of globin mRNA, such studies became feasible (*Verma et al.*, 1972; *Kacian et al.*, 1972; *Ross et al.*, 1972a). For the synthesis of DNA in this system the

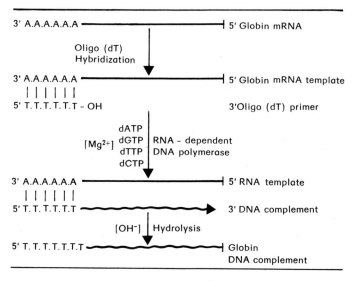

Fig. 38. Synthesis of the DNA complement of rabbit globin mRNA. (From *Ross et al.*, 1972a. Reproduced with the permission of the authors and the National Academy of Sciences, Washington.)

presence of a short homopolymer of thymidylate is essential (oligo(dT)$_{10-20}$) which primes initiation of reverse transcription by pairing with the poly(A)segment of globin mRNA (*see* p. 101). The formation of double stranded DNA can be prevented by addition of actinomycin D. The formed DNA complementary to globin mRNA template is denoted as cDNA (Fig. 38). Hybridization with labelled cDNA is then used for detection of molecules of globin mRNA (e.g. *Housman et al.* 1973; *Forget* and *Benz*, 1974; *Cann et al.*, 1974; *Gambino et al.*, 1974; *Gumerson* and *Williamson*, 1974; *Gazaryan et al.*, 1974; *Lanyon et al.*, 1975; *Skoultchi*, 1975). These methods are particularly suitable for assessment of the content of globin mRNA in erythroid cells during erythroid differentiation (*Gilmour et al.*, 1974; *Harrison et al.*, 1974; *Ramirez et al.*, 1975) and in erythroid cells of patients with thalassaemia. When using separate α- and β-globin mRNA as a template, complementary DNA can be prepared for the appropriate chain. By means of these cDNA corresponding to one chain only it is possible to assess the ratio of mRNA for α- and β-chains in the tested preparations of total mRNA for globin (*Housman et al.*, 1973; *Forget* and *Benz*, 1974). The hybridization method is very sensitive. The amount of tested mRNA can be as low as 10^{-9} g, while cell-free systems need 10^{-6} g for translation.

Characteristics of globin mRNA

As ensues from previous paragraphs, mRNA for globin was isolated from the reticulocytes of many animal species (e.g. *Chantrenne et al.*, 1967; *Schapira et al.*, 1968a; *Labrie*, 1969; *Lockard* and *Lingrel*, 1969; *Williamson et al.*, 1971; *Lingrel et al.*, 1971; *Borová et al.*, 1976) and man (e.g. *Benz* and *Forget*, 1971; *Nienhuis* and *Anderson*, 1971; *Metafora et al.*, 1972). Messenger RNA for globin was also isolated from nucleated cells of bone marrow (*Nienhuis* and *Anderson*, 1972; *Nienhuis et al.*, 1973; 1974) of the rabbit, sheep, goat and man and from the spleen of anaemic rabbits (*Nokin* and *Gautier*, 1973; *Nokin et al.*, 1975, *Fuchs*, *Borová* and *Poňka* − unpublished) and mice (*Cheng et al.*, 1974; *Fuchs et al.*, 1975). Isolated globin mRNA from these sources had, however, a lower biological activity when tested in a cell-free system than reticulocyte globin mRNA. The lower biological activity can perhaps be explained by some degree of degradation of globin mRNA during isolation, as bone marrow, and in particular the spleen, are tissues rich in ribonucleases.

The best preparations of globin mRNA migrate as a single diffuse band in polyacrylamide gels (e.g. *Lanyon et al.*, 1972; *Morrison et al.*, 1974; *Nokin et al.*, 1976). Separation of mRNA for α- and β-globin chains is made possible by polyacrylamide gel electrophoresis in the presence of formamide. It was revealed that the more slowly moving component contains primarily β-globin mRNA, whereas the faster moving component is enriched with α-globin mRNA (*Morrison et al.*, 1974; *Kazazian et al.*, 1974). Electrophoretic motility is, however, also influenced in a significant way by the length of the poly(A) sequence at the 3′-end of globin mRNA. The length of this segment in individual mRNA molecules differs markedly and this is reflected in

100

a different electrophoretic motility of mRNA molecules. Recently therefore serious doubts have been raised whether the electrophoretic technique can be used to separate mRNA molecules for α- and β-chains (*Nokin et al.*, 1976).

Data on the molecular weight of mRNA vary somewhat, depending on the method used for its estimation. From the electrophoretic mobility on polyacrylamide gel the molecular weight of globin mRNA was estimated to be roughly 200,000–230,000 daltons (*Labrie*, 1969; *Gaskill* and *Kabat*, 1971; *Pemberton et al.*, 1972; *Gould* and *Hamlyn*, 1973). A value of ca 170,000 daltons was obtained for mouse globin mRNA by analytical ultracentrifugation (*Williamson et al.*, 1971). By electrophoresis on 4% polyacrylamide in the presence of formamide the molecular weight of globin mRNA for the α-chain was estimated to be 202,000 daltons and for the β-chain 227,000 daltons (*Sherman et al.*, 1974). RNA molecules of this size must contain roughly 650 to 675 nucleotides. This is by as much as 200 nucleotides more than is needed for coding for of the α-chain (141 amino acids) and the β-chain (146 amino acids) of globin. This means that mRNA contains nucleotide sequences which are not translated.

This greater size of globin mRNA can be partly, though not completely, explained by the presence of the polyadenylic acid sequence [poly(A)] at 3′-terminus of the molecule (*Lim* and *Canellakis*, 1970; *Burr* and *Lingrel*, 1971). Recently it was revealed that globin mRNA has in the vicinity of the poly(A) segment a sequence ...-A-U-U-G-C-poly(A) (*Proudfoot* and *Brownlee*, 1974). Heterogeneity in the length of the poly(A) region has been observed in mouse α- and β-globin messenger RNAs. From the total poly(A) containing globin messenger RNA on Millipore filters — which retain only poly(A) segments longer than 50 nucleotides — only 30% globin mRNA are retained. Newly synthesized mRNA contains longer poly(A) sequences relative to older mRNAs and it seems thus that the length of the poly(A) segment is reduced by ageing of mRNA molecules (*Gorski et al.*, 1974; *Pemberton* and *Baglioni*, 1973). In several laboratories it was shown that translation of globin mRNA is also feasible in different cell-free systems after removal of poly(A) segments by the action of 3′-OH specific exonuclease which does not damage the remaining part of the mRNA molecule (*Humphries et al.*, 1974; *Williamson et al.*, 1974; *Huez et al.*, 1974; *Soreq et al.*, 1974). In cell-free systems it is, however, not possible to follow up long-term translation of globin mRNA and therefore some authors used *Xenopus* oocytes to compare the rate and extent of translation of both intact and poly(A)-free globin mRNA. The results revealed that during longer incubation periods the rate of globin synthesis with poly(A)-free mRNA is considerably lower than with native mRNA (*Huez et al.*, 1974). On the other hand, when the poly(A) sequence was resynthesized onto mRNA from which the poly(A) had been previously removed, the ability of the globin mRNA to control haemoglobin synthesis in oocytes was restored for a considerable period of time (Fig. 39) (*Huez et al.*, 1975; *see also Nudel et al.*, 1976). The poly(A) segment thus obviously appears to play an important role in maintaining the stability of globin mRNA. For this assumption direct evidence was provided recently by *Marbaix et al.* (1975) who measured the amount of mRNA molecules in oocytes using the technique of molecular hybridization. The same group of authors

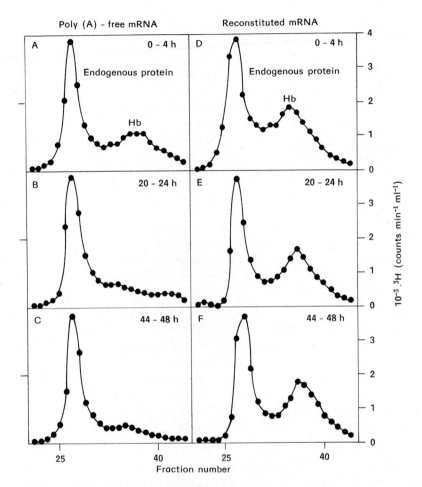

Fig. 39. Haemoglobin synthesis directed by rabbit globin poly(A)-free and reconstituted mRNA. 80 oocytes from a single *Xenopus laevis* female were microinjected with 50 nl each of mRNA aqueous solutions at 100 µg/ml. 40 of them received poly(A)-free mRNA (A, B, C) and the other 40 received reconstituted mRNA (D, E,F). Immediately (A, D), 20 h (B, E) and 44 h (C, F) after microinjection, 10 oocytes of each batch were incubated in 100 µl of Barth's medium containing mCi/ml of histidine-³H (50 Ci/nmol) at 19 °C for 4 h. At the end of the incubation, the oocytes were washed and homogenized. Cell debris were removed by low-speed centrifugation and the supernatant was analyzed by gel filtration on 1.70-cm Sephadex G-100 columns. Aliquots of the eluted fractions were removed and radioactivity measured in a toluene Triton X-100 mixture using a scintillation spectrometer. (From *Huez et al.*, 1975. Reproduced with the permission of the authors and Springer-Verlag, Heidelberg.)

demonstrated that poly(A)-free globin mRNA degradation in *Xenopus* oocytes depends on its translation (*Marbaix et al.*, 1976). All these results correspond to the fact that prokaryotic messenger RNA and histone mRNA which do not contain the poly(A) segment have a very short half-life.

The existence of the poly(A) segment, however, cannot completely explain the difference between the expected and actual length of globin mRNA. Very interesting evidence of the existence of a further normally untranslated region of globin mRNA was provided by clinical observations. There exist several haemoglobin variants with prolonged α-chains (e.g. Hb Constant Spring, ref. *Clegg et al.*, 1971b; *Milner et al.*, 1971 and Hb Wayne, ref. *Seid-Akhaven et al.*, 1972), or β-chains (e.g. Hb Cranston, ref. *Bunn et al.*, 1975). It was concluded that a mutation developed in or near the normal chain termination codon (*see* p. 121) which rendered possible the translation of normally untranslated sequences of the mRNA between the chain termination codon and the 3'-terminal poly(A). This hypothesis was recently confirmed: direct nucleotide sequence analysis of normal human globin mRNA (*Marotta et al.*, 1974; *Forget et al.*, 1974) has revealed predicted 3'-terminal nucleotide sequences of the α-chain mRNA which match amino acid sequences of the elongated portions of the variant α-chains. Similarly in normal messenger RNA for the human β-globin chain nucleotide sequences have been identified which can be matched with the amino acid sequence of the abnormally long segment of the β-chain of haemoglobin Cranston. The role of these additional segments has not been elucidated so far and the hypothesis was put forward that these segments represent a sequence of nucleotides important for combination with ribosomes (*Scherrer*, 1973).

Recent findings suggest that messenger RNAs from a wide variety of cellular and viral sources contain methylated constituents. *Perry* and *Scherrer* (1975) recently provided convincing evidence that the 9s globin mRNA produced in duck erythrocytes also contains "capped" 5'-terminal methylated sequences. This duck globin mRNA is relatively rich in sequences which contain two 2'-O-methyl nucleotides. The existence of 5'-terminal methylated sequences is important for template activity of globin mRNA. The β-elimination reaction — which removes the "capping nucleoside" (7-methylguanosine) and "uncaps" 5'-terminal sequences — impairs the template activity of globin mRNA. It seems that the removal of this 5'-nucleoside or even the demethylation of the 7-methylguanosine strongly lowered the affinity of the initiation site on the mRNA for the complex of the small ribosome sub-unit with methionyl-tRNA (*see* p. 115). It has been suggested that the loss of the 5'-terminal 7-methylguanosine occurs when mRNA ages (*Nokin et al.*, 1976).

Most of the biologically active mRNA for globin in erythroid cells is localized in cytoplasmic polyribosomes which synthesize globin. If purified polyribosomes are treated with EDTA or pyrophosphate, globin mRNA is released from polyribosomes bound to proteins as messenger ribonucleoprotein (mRNP) particles. The mRNP component sediments at 14s in sucrose gradients. Proteins of this component were isolated and characterized for the rabbit (*Lebleu et al.*, 1971). In all instances two main protein components were found. The molecular weights of the protein components were estimated to be 68,000 and 130,000 daltons in rabbits and 49,000 and 73,000 daltons in ducks. Originally it was assumed that these proteins serve in the binding of mRNA to its natural attachement site on the 40s ribosomal sub-unit (*Holder* and *Lingrel*, 1970). It must, however, be emphasized that no differences were revealed between 9 s mRNA and 14 s RNP with regard to their ability to stimulate protein synthesis in cell-free systems (*see* above). The only suggestion of a functional difference is in the binding of 14s mRNP to native 40s ribosomal sub-units which have been washed with deoxycholate. 9s mRNA does not bind with thus treated sub-units (*Lebleu et al.*, 1971; *Williamson*, 1973).

In addition to this polyribosomal mRNP there also exists cytoplasmic non-polyribosomal mRNP which contains in particular α-globin messenger activity (*see* p. 93). The function of proteins of this mRNP complex is not clear.

Biosynthesis of globin mRNA

It may be stated that the solution of problems associated with the biosynthesis of mRNA for globin are only in their initial phase. Nevertheless it is certain that in cells of higher organisms − and obviously also in erythroid cells which synthesize globin − the product of transcription of DNA is not mRNA with a molecular weight of 10^5 to 10^6 daltons (in the case of globin ca 2×10^5 daltons) but a much larger RNA (molecular weight as high as 10^7).

This RNA is found in mammalian nuclei and is called heterogeneous nuclear RNA (HnRNA), DNA-like RNA (*Georgiev et al.*, 1963), messenger-like RNA (*Scherrer* and *Marcaud*, 196᠄) and today there is a tendency to denote it as pre-messenger RNA (pre-mRNA). Recently the presence of sequences of messenger RNA for globin was unequivocally demonstrated in this high-molecular pre-mRNA. Duck HnRNA contains globin mRNA sequences detectable by hybridization of HnRNA with globin cDNA (*Imaiz ᠄mi et al.*, 1973; *Scherrer*, 1973). Similarly HnRNA from mouse erytroblasts contains haemoglobin mesenger sequences. Injection of this HnRNA into *Xenopus* oocytes induces in these cells synthesis of mouse globin (*Williamson et al.*, 1973). High molecular newly formed RNA can be considered a mediator between DNA and true messenger RNA. The non-coding part of high-molecular pre-messenger RNA does not necessarily imply senseless sequences but rather sequences which have a certain programme. It is assumed that pre-messenger RNA contains not only the transcribed DNA code but also the programme for its subsequent fate. *Scherrer* (1973) suggests for this part of the molecule of pre-messenger RNA the term programming sequences. Information provided by this code would determine not only the transcription of messenger RNA but also post-transcription regulation and the fate of the given information in time and space during its genesis, passage into the cytoplasm and translation on polyribosomes.

Landhoff et al. (1975) recently isolated from rabbit erythroid cells pre-mRNA molecules sedimenting at > 45 s and investigated them by electron microscopy. In some of the pre-mRNA molecules a characteristic condensed structure was observed at one end strikingly resembling the structure of the mRNA molecule. From previous studies of *Coutelle et al.* (1970) and *Georgiev et al.* (1972) it appears that mRNA sequences are located at the 3'-end of HnRNA (pre-mRNA).

Poly(A) sequence of mature RNA is not transcribed directly from the cell DNA but is added to mRNA by a post-transcription mechanism (*Darnell et al.*, 1973; *Mansbridge et al.*, 1974). It is possible that addition of the poly(A) sequence is associated with the maturation and processing of the HnRNA and it is beyond doubt that poly(A) plays a very important role in the stability of mRNA (*see* above).

Little is known so far about the process by which globin mRNA is transported from the nucleus into the cytoplasm. mRNA is not transported into the cytoplasm in a free form but in association with proteins as messenger ribonucleoprotein particles (*Williamson et al.*, 1973).

The elucidation of mechanisms by which transcription of globin mRNA in erythroid cells is controlled is only in its earliest stages. Non-differentiated precursors of erythroid cells (erythroid committed stem cells or erythropoietin sensitive cells) evidently do not synthesize globin mRNA. RNA synthesis for globin is initiated only after contact of these cells with the humoral inductor erythropoietin (*Gross* and *Goldwasser*, 1971; *Terada et al.*, 1972) (*see* p. 152). The exact mechanism of action at the molecular level still awaits complete elucidation, nevertheless it is clear that in erythroid cells transcriptional units containing the globin structural genes are activated (by unpacking and uncoiling of the chromatin fibre) which renders possible specific expression of globin genes (i.e. globin mRNA synthesis). Direct evidence was produced that chromatin isolated from erythroid cells of the duck (*Axel et al.*, 1973), foetal mouse liver (*Gilmour* and *Paul*, 1973; *Gilmour et al.*, 1975) and the rabbit (*Steggles et al.*, 1974; *Wilson et al.*, 1975) can be transcribed in an *in vitro* system into globin specific mRNA sequences in the presence of DNA-dependent RNA polymerase. Chromatin from duck and rabbit livers or mouse brain is, however, not transcribed in this *in vitro* system into globin mRNA, although these cells contain globin genes in their DNA. For transcription of globin mRNA the presence of chromosomal proteins is essential, as purified DNA from erythroid cells is not transcribed (*Wilson et al.*, 1975). It seems that non-histone proteins of chromatin are specific factors controlling the transcription of genes. Acidic proteins derived from erythroid cell chromatin control the transcription of the globin gene from non-erythroid chromatin (*Gilmour*, 1973; *Gilmour et al.*, 1975). Recent experiments indicate that haem might be involved in the formation of globin mRNA (*Dabney* and *Beaudet*, 1976; *Ross* and *Sautner*, 1976; *Poňka et al.*, 1977a). This may represent a mechanism by which the transcription of globin message is quantitatively controlled and coordinated with the rate of haem synthesis (cf. p. 135).

However, numerous questions pertaining to the mechanism of transcription, its regulation and to the initiation of DNA template activation in erythropoietin sensitive cells and the activity of globin DNA templates during the cell cycle and the subsequent maturation of erythroid cells remain open. The possibility must also be considered that globin mRNA can be synthesized independently of DNA template because the enzyme RNA-dependent RNA polymerase was isolated from erythroid cells which is able to synthesize RNA when primed by cytoplasmic globin mRNA (*Downey et al.*, 1973).

Transfer RNA

Transfer RNA (4s) accomplishes the transfer of amino acids to the proper site in the messenger RNA template as it can recognize the codons on the mRNA. For each of the 20 naturally occurring amino acids there must be at least one or more RNAs (the code is degenerated) but each tRNA type functions only for one amino acid. There is base pairing between some of the bases which results in a "clover leaf" pattern of tRNA. The 3′-end of the chain always terminates in the CCA sequence and the 5′-end terminates with guanine. The amino acid is attached at the 3′-end forming the aminoacyl-tRNA. The so-called anti-codon contains three unpaired bases capable of recognizing the complementary bases in mRNA. This is the most specific end of the molecule and the one which reads the message. In tRNA there is also a ribosome recognition site which is common to all these molecules and another site related to the recognition of the specific amino acid activating enzyme.

Prior to binding to RNA every amino acid is activated by reacting with ATP to form aminoacyl adenylate. A specific amino acid activating enzyme for every amino acid is required. Activating enzymes deprived of haemoglobin and RNA were demonstrated in reticulocytes by *Allen* and *Schweet* in 1962. The enzyme-bound activated amino acid is then transferred to tRNA (a transacylation) to form aminoacyl-tRNA. The enzyme responsible for this reaction is called aminoacyl-tRNA synthetase.

Haemoglobin can be formed on polyribosomes of rabbit reticulocytes by using tRNA prepared from *Escherichia coli* (*von Ehrenstein* and *Lipmann*, 1961; *von Ehrenstein et al.*, 1963; *Galizzi*, 1969), from guinea-pig liver (*Bishop et al.*, 1961), yeasts (*Weisblum et al.*, 1967), mouse tumours and normal mouse liver (*Muschinski et al.*, 1970). These experiments provide evidence that the tRNAs mentioned can be used by proteosynthetic components from another quite remote organism.

Recently several authors have presented data showing that within the reticulocyte the level of tRNA species for a given amino acid is correlated with the relative content of the amino acid in haemoglobin (*Smith* and *McNamara*, 1971; *Litt* and *Kabat*, 1972; *Smith*, 1975). This specialization of the tRNA content for haemoglobin synthesis was demonstrated in rabbit, sheep and human reticulocytes. The investigations using sheep reticulocytes are particularly convincing. When some sheep are made anaemic, they synthesize a haemoglobin with a β-chain of abnormal amino acid composition.

106

The relative amounts of different tRNAs are correlated with the amino acid composition of the sheep haemoglobins which are being synthesized (*Litt* and *Kabat*, 1972). However, there are exceptions to this relationship. In rabbit reticulocytes there is a great excess of methionine tRNA compared with the methionine content in rabbit haemoglobin even if we take into account the labile methionine residue at the amino-terminus of each sub-unit chain (*see* p. 114). Conversely leucine tRNA is scarce, compared with the abundance of leucine in haemoglobin. Similarly a certain type of sheep reticulocytes which do not require any isoleucine for haemoglobin synthesis contain measurable amounts of isoleucine tRNA (*Litt* and *Kabat*, 1972). Excess of some tRNA could be explained by the indispensibility of these tRNA for the synthesis of non-haemoglobin proteins in reticulocytes. Excess methionine in tRNA may perhaps be the manifestation of a certain adaptational mechanism by means of which an adequate non-limiting amount of tRNA important for the initiation of the chain is ensured for the cell. On the other hand, relative deficiency of a certain tRNA could influence, and perhaps regulate, the rate of elongation of the globin chain (*see also* p. 127). It seems thus probable that the levels of the tRNA species in the reticulocytes are subject to control by the amino acid composition of haemoglobin. A certain type of feedback seems to be involved which is implemented either at the level of tRNA synthesis, maturation or degradation.

RIBOSOMES AND GLOBIN SYNTHESIS

Ribosomes are ultramicroscopic biochemical "machines" on which, during interaction of mRNA and tRNA, a polypeptide chain is synthesized. The ribosome is not merely an inert frame joining together mRNA and tRNA in the correct way, but many of its proteins play various parts in the synthesis of the peptide chain. Ribosomes are the site of protein synthesis in all cells from bacteria to mammalian cells and although these cells are very remote, their ribosomes have basically a similar composition and shape. The function of all ribosomes in all organisms is the same and no other biochemical protein producing system is known. Ribosomes are nucleoprotein particles. In mammalian cells — and also erythroid cells — they are either free in the cytoplasm or bound to membrane structures.

Ribosome structure

The ribosome has a roughly spherical shape and is made up of two sub-units, one roughly twice the size of the other. In *Escherichia coli* the intact ribosome (70s) consists of sub-units with sedimentation coefficients of 50s and 30s. In reticulocytes, similarly as in other eukaryotic cells, the corresponding sedimentation coefficients are considerably greater: the 80s ribosome is made up of a 60s and 40s sub-unit. Table 12 summarizes our knowledge on properties of ribosomes from rabbit reticulocytes (*Cox* and *Bonanou*, 1969).

Table 12

Properties of rabbit reticulocyte ribosomes

Property	Value	Reference
Molecular weight	$4.0 \cdot 10^6 - 4.1 \cdot 10^6$	*Dintzis et al.* (1958)
RNA (g)/protein (g) ratio	1 : 1	*Dintzis et al.* (1958)
$S^{\circ}_{20,w}$	80 ± 2 s (ribosome) 60 ± 2 s (larger subparticle) 40 ± 2 s (smaller subparticle)	
(η)	8 ml/g	*Dintzis et al.* (1958)
Partial specific volume	0.63 ml/g	*Dintzis et al.* (1958)
Frictional ratio (f/f$_o$)	1.72	*Dintzis et al.* (1958)
Dimensions from electron microscopy	250 Å . 175 Å (negative staining) 200 Å . 155 Å (positive staining)	*Mathias et al.* (1964) *Mathias et al.* (1964)
Radius of gyration	108 Å	*Dibble* and *Dintzis* (1960)
Diameter in solution	340 Å	*Dintzis et al.* (1958)
Axial ratio	1 : 1	*Dintzis et al.* (1958)
Behaviour in solution	Compact particle	*Inouye et al.* (1963)
Molecular weight of RNA	$3 \cdot 10^4, 0.5 \cdot 10^6 - 0.64 \cdot 10^6, 1.5 \cdot 10^6$	*Bachvaroff* and *Tongur* (1966) *Cox* and *Arnstein* (1963) *Hunt* (1970)
Molecular weight of polypeptide	32 proteins were identified in the 40 s subunit; m.w. 8,000–39,000 39 proteins were identified in the 60 s subunit; m.w. 9,000–58,000	*Howard et al.* (1975)
X-ray diffraction	45–50 Å reflexion	*Langridge* (1963)

(Adapted from *Cox* and *Bonanou*, 1969.)

Proteins. Each ribosome consists of many proteins which can be divided into three main groups: (1) Structural ribosomal proteins which remain associated with ribosomes even after their thorough purification. Structural ribosomal proteins are arranged in such a way that they render possible specific binding as well as catalytic functions of ribosomes. (2) Not quite pure ribosome preparations contain proteins which are essential for complete biological activity of ribosomes. These proteins comprise initiation factors (*see* p. 117) and the dissociation factor (*see* p. 122). (3)

Crude ribosome preparations contain moreover various enzymes which are not related to the structure or function of ribosomes (*Spirin* and *Gavrilova*, 1969).

Proteins of mammalian ribosomes are characterized by a high content of basic amino acids (*Mathias* and *Williamson*, 1964). A large sub-unit contains $40-60$ proteins with molecular weights between 8,000 and 57,000 daltons and 30 to 40 proteins present in a small sub-unit which have a molecular weight of 6,000 to 39,000 daltons (*King et al.*, 1971; *Howard et al.*, 1975). Several ribosomal proteins in rabbit reticulocytes are phosphoproteins (*Kabat*, 1970, 1971; *Martini* and *Gould*, 1973). The phosphate groups turn over within the cells, as was demonstrated by the labelling of ribosomal proteins in reticulocytes incubated with orthophosphate-^{32}P. It was suggested that the phosphorylation of one protein on the large ribosomal sub-unit inactivates the ribosomes which then cannot participate in the ribosome cycle of protein synthesis.

Ribosomal RNA. Every ribosomal sub-unit contains one simple RNA chain which serves as a frame for the attachment of ribosomal proteins. The secondary structure of ribosomal RNA (rRNA) determines the shape of the sub-unit. The sedimentation coefficient of the small RNA sub-unit is 18s and of the large sub-unit 28s. 18s ribosomal RNA from reticulocytes has a molecular weight of 0.64×10^6 daltons, the 28s sub-unit 1.5×10^6 daltons (*Hunt*, 1970). The large sub-unit of bacterial as well as mammalian ribosomes contains yet other species of RNA with a sedimentation coefficient of 5 s (*Christman* and *Goldstein*, 1969; *Zehavi-Willner*, 1970; *Zehavi-Willner* and *Danon*, 1972).

Recently a direct formerly not assumed function in protein synthesis was ascribed to 18s ribosomal RNA. It was found that exogenous liver or reticulocyte 18s ribosomal RNA potentiates translation of 9s globin mRNA and renders it at·least ten times more efficient. It has been suggested that a specific reversible association develops between the initiation region of mRNA and a region of 18s rRNA (which is accessible on the surface of 40s ribosomal sub-units). According to this concept thus 9s globin mRNA is an inactive molecule which is normally potentiated by this specific reversible base pairing (*Kabat*, 1975).

The intricate questions pertaining to the structure of ribosomes as a whole are resolved mainly by using methods focused on the secondary structure of rRNA inside the ribosome. *Cox* and *Bonanou* (1969) endeavoured to produce a speculative model of ribosomes of rabbit reticulocytes based on data of various workers. Interaction between proteins of sub-units and rRNA loops, which have the shape of a hairpin, is assumed. The ribonucleoprotein thread of the large sub-unit forms a horseshoe and this conformation may be maintained by 5s RNA. The small sub-unit fits as a cap on the larger sub-unit. Both particles combined form a hollow cylinder. Messenger RNA is probably bound on the inner surface of the smaller sub-unit. This suggestion is in agreement with the observation that polyribosomes dissociate directly into sub-units without the formation of ribosomes as intermediates. The polypeptide chain probably grows from the channel between the two sub-units. This view is supported by the finding that the portion of the newly growing chain containing 30–50 amino acid residues is shielded from a proteolytic attack (*Rich et al.*, 1966).

To maintain the structural integrity of the ribosome ions of bivalent metals, in particular magnesium ions, are essential. Mg^{2+} ions are needed in ribosomes not only for the mutual combination of the two parts but also to preserve the structure of sub-units (*Spirin* and *Gavrilova*, 1969). It is also well known that monovalent ions exert a stabilizing action on the secondary structure of RNA. K^+-deficient ribosomes from reticulocytes are abnormally sensitive to ribonuclease (*Näslund* and *Hultin*, 1970; 1971). It must, however, be mentioned that a high KCl concentration causes dissociation of ribosomes into sub-units (*Yang et al.*, 1968; *see* p. 111).

The role of polyribosomes

The role of ribosomes (or according to the original term microsomes) in protein synthesis (*Littlefield et al.*, 1955) and also in haemoglobin synthesis (*Rabinovitz* and *Olson*, 1956) was discovered more than 20 years ago. The discovery that the site of haemoglobin synthesis *in vivo* is not a single ribosome but a group of ribosomes (*Warner et al.*, 1962; *Marks et al.*, 1962; *Warner et al.*, 1963; *Gierer*, 1963) was made only in 1962. At that time it was demonstrated that after incubation of reticulocytes with amino acids labelled with ^{14}C those ribosomal fractions are labelled most actively which have a considerably greater sedimentation coefficient than the sedimentation coeficient of single ribosomes (*Warner et al.*, 1962; *Marks et al.*, 1962). In addition *Warner et al.* (1962) presented electron micrographs indicating that protein synthesis within the reticulocyte occurs in a multiple ribosomal structure containing 5 ribosomes. These structures denoted as polyribosomes or also polysomes (170s) were broken down into individual ribosomes (76s) by the action of ribonuclease. It was therefore suggested that the ribosomal units are held together by mRNA.

The above facts led to the formulation of the concept of polyribosome function. This concept assumes that individual ribosomes in the polysome move along mRNA simultaneously with the growth of the polypeptide chain and become detached at the end of mRNA with the completion of the chain (*Goodman* and *Rich*, 1963). According to this model synthesis of the polypeptide chain begins by the addition of the ribosome to mRNA. Later it was revealed (*see* p. 112) that monoribosomes are not directly involved in the ribosomal cycle but ribosomal sub-units directly exchange with ribosomes in the polyribosome pool (*see* Fig. 41).

The general concept of the polyribosome function is still valid and is supported by various experiments among which we shall mention only the most interesting. Amino acids are not distributed evenly in globin chains and this fact was used by some workers to test the function of polyribosomes in rabbit reticulocytes. It is well known that haemoglobin synthesis takes place from the NH_2-terminal amino acid to the COOH-terminal amino acid (*Dintzis*, 1961; *Naughton* and *Dintzis* 1962;

110

Rychlík and *Šorm,* 1962). Theoretically the deficiency of a single amino acid which is localized near the N-terminal end only should not permit the ribosome to pass this point. The translation rate beyond the site of deficiency should, however, be quite normal which naturally would lead to disaggregation of polyribosomes. On the other hand, the deficiency of an amino acid which is localized near the C-terminus only should lead to the accumulation of ribosomes on the mRNA molecule. *Hori et al.* (1967) actually provided evidence that the selective deficiency of tryptophan which is near the amino-terminus of rabbit haemoglobin is associated with disaggregation of polyribosomes in reticulocytes.

In rabbit erythroid cells the codon for isoleucine is located near the proximal end of mRNA for α-chains and near the distal end of mRNA for β-chains (*see* p. 93). Inhibition of globin synthesis by O-methylthreonine, which is an isoleucine antagonist, is associated with marked changes in polyribosomes. *Hori* and *Rabinovitz* (1968) explained these changes by the fact that polyribosomes which synthesize α-chains diminish in size while polyribosomes where β-chains are formed, increase in size. *Kazazian* and *Freedman* (1968) confirmed this assumption by direct analysis of nascent chains on small and large polysomes. Fig. 34 illustrates schematically changes in polysomes synthesizing α- and β-chains in rabbit reticulocytes incubated with an isoleucine antagonist.

Similarly the polyribosome model can be readily tested by using specific inhibitors of initiation (NaF, haem deficit). Inhibited initiation of the globin chain is associated with disaggregation of polysomes in reticulocytes. If, however, at the same time an inhibitor of elongation is added (e.g. cycloheximide) which inhibits the growth of the nascent globin and "freezes" the movement of ribosomes along mRNA template, the dissociation of reticulocyte polyribosomes can be prevented (*Godchaux et al.,* 1967).

Various changes in ribosomes are caused by incubation of reticulocytes with iron chelates (which induce intracellular haem deficiency) or with haemin. These results are discussed in more detail in the chapter on the role of haem in globin synthesis (*see* p. 129).

The role of sub-units

The reticulocyte lysate contains in addition to polyribosomes and monoribosomes also ribosomal sub-units (*Bishop,* 1965; 1966a; 1966b). Native ribosomal sub-units are much more active during the synthesis of the chain than whole ribosomes and thus it was concluded that sub-units are active components during the initiation of polypeptide synthesis (*Bishop,* 1965).

Ribosomal sub-units can be prepared with higher yields, using various methods. Ribosomal sub-particles may be prepared from ribosomes treated with EDTA (*Gould et al.,* 1966), with a high KCl concentration (e.g. *Yang et al.,* 1968; *Hamada et al.,* 1968; *Godin et al.,* 1969; *Bonanou* and *Arnstein,* 1969; *Cohen,* 1970 − see

Fig. 40), from ribosomes exposed to pyrophosphate (*Holder* and *Lingrel*, 1970) or from reticulocytes incubated at low temperatures (*Fuhr et al.*, 1971). The preparation of sub-units by centrifugation in a high (0.5 M) KCl concentration is very popular; however, by this treatment ribosomal sub-particles are deprived of initiating factors and are not active in the protein synthesis in the cell-free system. The activity is restored by adding ribosomal wash proteins or initiating factors (*see* Fig. 40).

The importance and role of sub-units in globin synthesis were demonstrated by several experimental approaches. First, addition of sub-units to the cell-free system from reticulocytes markedly stimulates amino acid incorporation into proteins. Secondly, disaggregation of polysomes caused by tryptophan deficiency is associated with a rise in the level of free ribosomal sub-units (*Freedman* and *Rabinovitz*, 1970). This finding can be explained by the fact that monoribosomes are released from polyribosomes after termination of every translation cycle and dissociate into sub-units (*Colombo et al.*, 1968). The third experimental approach was used by *Adamson et al.*, (1969b). These authors labelled polyribosomes with ^{32}P and added the labelled polyribosomes to a cell-free system which contained unlabelled components of the ribosomal system. During incubation the radioactivity of polysomes declined and at the same time the radioactivity of small and large ribosomal sub-units increased. Monoribosomes were, however, not labelled. After reaching a dynamic equilibrium, the specific activities of sub-units and polyribosomes were equal (*Howard et al.*, 1970a). These results indicate that both sub-units are exchanging with polyribosomes and that the majority of monoribosomes are not directly involved in the ribosomal cycle in the cell-free system.

Membrane-bound ribosomes

Burka et al. (1967a) found that part of the reticulocyte RNA is in the cell membrane. The sedimentation coefficients of the membrane bound RNAs — 18 s, 28 s and 4 s — indicate that the reticulocyte membrane contains rRNA as well as tRNA (*Burka et al.*, 1967b).

Bulova and *Burka* (1970) suggested that membrane-bound ribosomes serve for the synthesis of high-molecular non-haemoglobin proteins, while globin is synthesized preferentially on free ribosomes, However, other workers (*Lodish*, 1973; *Woodward et al.*, 1973) did not find evidence for this specialization of reticulocyte ribosomes and demonstrated that both free and membrane bound ribosomes synthesize globin and non-globin proteins equally well.

Function of the active ribosomal complex

The mechanism of formation of the globin chain has been elucidated to a considerable extent due to many years' effort on the part of research workers in many laboratories. It may be said that during investigations of globin synthesis basic knowledge was assembled concerning the mechanism of protein synthesis in eukaryotes and all hitherto assembled knowledge suggests that the mechanism of protein formation is identical in all eukaryotic cells. The basic mechanisms of protein formation are, however, very similar throughout nature, in eukaryotes and prokaryotes, and differ only in certain details (*Lucas-Lenard* and *Lipmann*, 1971) which will be emphasized. The formation of the globin chain involving the interaction of globin messenger RNA, transfer RNA and ribosomes proceeds through three consecutive stages: chain initiation, elongation and termination. In the subsequent paragraphs we shall try to summarize the present views on these events. More detailed reviews concerning protein synthesis (*Lucas-Bernard* and *Lippman*, 1971; *Haselkorn* and *Rothman-Denes*, 1973) and globin synthesis (*Benz* and *Forget*, 1974) may be found in the papers quoted.

Initiation of the globin chain

Globin messenger RNA has a rather complex structure and moreover the sequence determining the primary structure of the globin chain contains further untranslated sequences (*see* p. 101). For the correct translation of the message laid down in the messenger RNA it is essential to commence the reading of the message at the correct site; this is ensured by the process called initiation.

Before 1970 it seemed that the initiation of globin synthesis is quite different from initiation of protein synthesis in bacterial systems, i.e. originally evidence of the existence of an initiating amino acid was lacking. Subsequently the initiating amino acid was discovered but certain differences in the initiation of the two systems nevertheless exist. In bacteria protein synthesis is initiated by binding of mRNA with a small ribosomal sub-unit. Then formylmethionyl-tRNA combines with the initiation codon of the mRNA molecule (AUG) and the complex is joined by a large ribosomal sub-unit. The first amino acid (formylmethionine) is subsequently deformylated and completely removed from the polypeptide chain. The process of initiation requires the participation of three initiation factors: IF-1, IF-2, IF-3. IF-2 directs the binding of the formylmethionyl-tRNA to the small ribosomal sub-unit and this binding is stabilized by IF-1. IF-3 assists in the ribosomal binding of mRNA.

Initiation of globin synthesis by means of methionyl-tRNA

Globin biosynthesis takes place from the N-terminal amino acid by consecutive addition of amino acid residues (*Dintzis*, 1961). The N-terminal amino acid of the α- and β-chain of rabbit and human haemoglobin is valine. All experiments made before 1969 seemed to suggest that the formation of globin chains is initiated by valine which is the N-terminal amino acid (e.g. *Rahaminoff* and *Arnstein*, 1968; *Gonano* and *Baglioni*, 1969). At that time it was generally assumed that the initiation of chain production in eukaryotic cells differed completely from the process in bacteria (*Clark* and *Marcker*, 1965, 1966).

Later, however, several groups of workers proved more or less independently that the synthesis of globin chains is initiated by methionine incorporation into the N-terminal position (*Wilson* and *Dintzis*, 1969; 1970; *Jackson* and *Hunter*, 1970; *Yoshida et al.*, 1970). *Wilson* and *Dintzis* (1970) demonstrated that chain initiation in haemoglobin synthesis involved the attachement of some group to the N-terminal valine. Analysis of tryptic peptides of nascent chains bound to ribosomes revealed that a small proportion of N-terminal peptide contained methionine at the N-terminus. The elegant and conclusive experiments of *Jackson* and *Hunter* (1970) are also worth mentioning. Rabbit reticulocytes were incubated with NaF, which prevented new chain initiation, while protein formation which had began before addition of NaF was completed. Thus the ribosomes were "synchronized" in the pre-initiation stage of the globin chain. The authors rendered the initiation of new chains possible by removal of NaF but arrested further growth of the chain by addition of another inhibitor, sparsomycin. It is obvious that in the presence of sparsomycin only very short peptides must be formed. *Jackson* and *Hunter* were able to demonstrate that in these short peptides only methionine and valine were present. The initiating methionine is then removed during subsequent stages of chain growth. The cleavage occurs probably when the nascent chain has a length of 15–30 amino acids (*Yoshida et al.*, 1970; *Yoshida* and *Lin*, 1972).

The above experiments suggested that the initiator tRNA for globin synthesis is methionyl-tRNA. Experiments performed with reticulocytes confirmed this assumption and revealed that a special initiating tRNA, i.e. methionyl-tRNA$_f$* takes methionine to a N-terminal position of nascent haemoglobin chains (*Housman et al.*, 1970; *Bhaduri et al.*, 1970; *Gupta et al.*, 1970; *Anderson* and *Schafritz*, 1971). Authors of all these investigations were able to show that methionyl-tRNA$_f$ recognizes the initiation AUG codon and thus initiates synthesis of the globin chain. On the other hand, methionyl-tRNA$_m$** conveys methionine for the internal position of the polypeptide chain. The basis of this mechanism recognizing the initiation codon is not clear so far. As will ensue from the subsequent text, in the process of initiation a very complex structure made up of methionyl-tRNA$_f$ bound to a small ribosomal sub-unit (40 s) together with nucleotide triphosphate and initiation factors participate. It is possible that the tridimensional structure of this complex identifies the initiating AUG codon and differentiates it from inner AUG codons of mRNA which determine methionine in the globin chain. It is possible that for the correct interaction of this complex at the 5'-terminal end of mRNA, untranslated nucleotide sequences localized there are more important than the AUG codon *per se* (*Schreier* and *Staehlin*, 1973d).

Initiation of globin synthesis in reticulocytes — similar to initiation of protein synthesis in other eukaryotic cells — differs markedly in one respect from the in-

---

*Methionyl-tRNA$_f$ can be formylated by transformylase from *Escherichia coli*.
**Cannot be formylated.

itiation process in prokaryotes. The bacterial ribosome needs N-formylmethionyl-tRNA for the initiation of protein synthesis. Globin synthesis, on the other hand, starts with methionine which is not formylated. The N-formylmethionyl residue can be incorporated into globin chains but formylated methionine cannot be removed from the nascent polypeptide chain (*Housman et al.*, 1970). The explanation may be that reticulocyte aminopeptidase which normally removes methionine from the growing peptide chain is unable to cleave formylmethionine. After addition of artificially formylated formylmethionyl-tRNA$_f$ to the globin synthesizing system, marked inhibition of protein formation can be observed. It may therefore be concluded that the structure of nascent chains affects the rate of protein synthesis.

Views on the exact order of events in the formation of the initiation complex (i.e. the complex of both sub-units combined with globin mRNA and methionyl-tRNA$_f$) developed gradually. Originally it seemed that the first step in the initiation is the binding of the small sub-unit of the ribosome (40s) to globin mRNA (*Hoerz* and *McCarty*, 1969; *Lebleu et al.*, 1970; *Heywood* and *Thompson*, 1971; *Pragnell* and *Arnstein*, 1970). These views were based on the observation that in the absence of initiation tRNA, mRNA is bound to a small sub-unit, depending on the initiation factor and that under favourable conditions a complete initiation complex may be formed. In 1973, however, *Schreier* and *Staehelin* published an observation that in the absence of mRNA methionyl-tRNA$_f$ is bound to a small ribosomal sub-unit in the presence of two initiating factors (IF-E$_2$ and IF-E$_3$). At the same time *Hunt, Jackson* and their co-workers described that reticulocyte lysates contain 40s methionyl-tRNA$_f$ complexes which are intermediates in the initiation of protein synthesis before the involvement of messenger RNA (*Darnbrough et al.*, 1973). The work of both groups thus supports the following model of the formation of the initiation complex during globin synthesis:

(1)   40s + met-tRNA$_f$ $\rightleftharpoons$ 40s/met-tRNA$_f$ complex

(2)   40s met-tRNA$_f$ + mRNA $\longrightarrow$ 40s/met-tRNA$_f$/mRNA complex

(3)   40s/met-tRNA$_f$/mRNA + 60s $\longrightarrow$ 80s/met-tRNA$_f$/mRNA complex (*see* Fig. 41).

It must be mentioned that even before the association of methionyl-tRNA$_f$ with the small sub-unit a complex of methionyl-tRNA$_f$ with GTP is formed in the presence of a certain factor (probably IF-E$_2$) which may be identical with IF-MP (*see* below).

The sequence of events in the initial stages of initiation is thus reversed, compared with initiation in bacterial systems. This reverse sequence of events during initiation and absence of the formyl group on the N-terminal initiation amino acid are two basic differences by which initiation in eukaryotes differs from a similar process in prokaryotic systems.

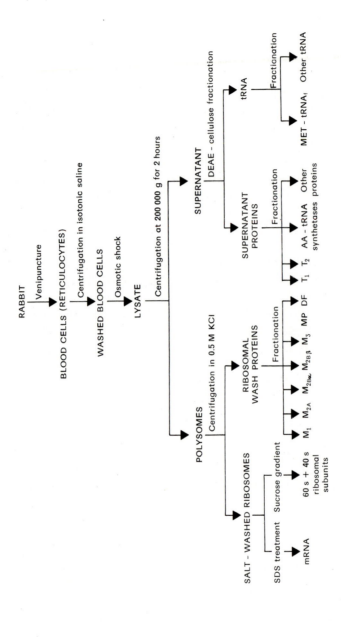

Fig. 40. Flow chart for the preparation of the fractionated cell-free protein synthesis system from rabbit reticulocytes. For details *see Gilbert and Anderson* (1970; *Shafritz and Anderson* (1970). (From *Anderson et al.*, 1975. Reproduced with the permission of the authors and Wistar Institute Press, Philadelphia.)

116

Initiation factors of reticulocyte ribosomes

Miller and *Schweet* (1968) were the first to find that washing reticulocyte ribosomes with a KCl solution removes from ribosomes the fraction which is essential for *de novo* haemoglobin synthesis (i.e. repeated initiation of new globin chains in cell-free systems) and which, as was demonstrated later, contains initiation factors. Nowadays this"ribosomal salt wash" is commonly used as initial material for the isolation of initiation factors (Fig. 40).

The present position with regard to the number and exact role of initiation factors in the synthesis of globin chains is somewhat confusing and so far there is no uniform nomenclature of initiation factors. *Anderson* and co-workers have used the term M (mammalian) and more recently IF-M, and *Schreier* and *Staehelin* use the symbol IF-E (E, eukaryote). *Anderson et al.* (e.g. *Prichard et al.*, 1970; *Shafritz et al.*, 1972; *Prichard* and *Anderson*, 1974; *Merrick et al.*, 1974; 1975; *Safer et al.*, 1975; *Filipowicz et al.*, 1976) isolated so far from rabbit reticulocytes six initiation factors: IF-MP, IF-M$_1$, IF-M$_{2A}$, IF-M$_{2B\alpha}$, IF-M$_{2B\beta}$ and IF-M$_3$. *Staehelin* and *Schreier* originally purified four initiation factors from rabbit reticulocytes: IF-E$_{1,2,3,4}$ (*Schreier* and *Staehelin* 1973c,d) but more recently *Staehelin et al.* (1975) reported the requirement for six factors in eukaryotic initiation. Comparison of the results of these two working teams is, however, so far impossible as different isolation and assay procedures were used. Nevertheless it seems that IF-E$_3$ resembles or is identical with IF-M$_3$ described by *Anderson et al.* Moreover, factor IF-E$_2$ described by *Schreier* and *Staehelin* seems to be identical with IF-MP of *Anderson*. Initiation factors were also isolated in other laboratories. Some seem to be identical with those of *Anderson et al.* (*Heywood*, 1970a; *Heywood* and *Thompson*, 1971), others are similar or different (*Chen et al.*, 1972; *Gupta et al.*, 1971, 1973, 1974; *Gupta* and *Aerni*, 1973; *Woodley et al.*, 1972; *Cashion* and *Stanley*, 1974).

Due to lack of uniformity in the nomenclature of factors, isolation and assay conditions, it is rather difficult to obtain an accurate idea on the participation of individual factors in the complex process of initiation. As has been suggested above, IF-E$_2$ (or IF-MP) binds free methionyl-tRNA$_f$ and GTP to form the initial complex during the initiation process. Then the 40s sub-unit is added and this complex with IF-M$_3$, IF-M$_{2A}$, IF-M$_{2B}$ and mRNA is joined by the 60s sub-unit to form 80s initiation complex (*Filipowicz et al.*, 1976) (Fig. 41). Originally it seemed that for the specific addition of globin mRNA a specific reticulocyte factor (IF-M$_3$) is essential (*Heywood* 1970; *Prichard et al.*, 1970; 1971; *Nudel et al.*, 1973; *Wigle*, 1973; *Lebleu et al.*, 1972) but no similar factor from other cells. Evidence was also submitted that there are factors which preferentially stimulate translation of α- or β-chain specific mRNA (*Fuhr* and *Natta*, 1972; *Hall* and *Arnstein*, 1973). As was emphasized, however, in the section dealing with globin mRNA (*see* p. 96), translation of globin mRNA in many heterologous systems without any special requirement for initiation factors proved possible. It is thus obvious that there is no specific initiation factor which is absolutely essential for translation. This is also in keeping with the recent finding that isolated liver IF-M$_3$ is equally active in promoting globin mRNA directed globin synthesis, as a similar initiation factor of reticulocyte origin (*Picciano et al.*, 1973). Adding of the 60s sub-unit to the complex 40s/met-tRNA$_f$/mRNA seems to require factor IF-E$_4$. This stage calls for GTP hydrolysis and perhaps some role is also played by IF-M$_{2A}$ which is capable of catalyzing ribosome-dependent GTP hydrolysis.

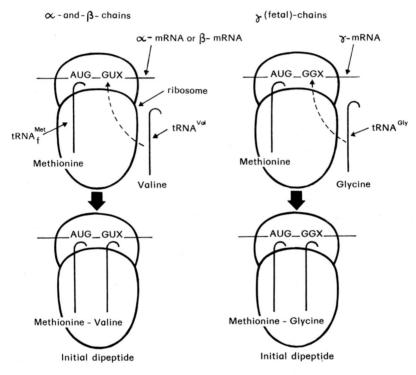

Fig. 41. Schematic representation of the initiation of human globin synthesis. (From *Anderson*, 1974. Reproduced with the permission of the author and the New York Academy of Sciences, New York.)

The formation of an initiation complex thus requires not only ribosome precursors (i.e. free ribosomal sub-units, mRNA and tRNA) but also other additional factors. This process is quite harmonious and it is not clear whether it takes place in the order outlined above or whether some processes take place simultaneously. It is again obvious that the process of initiation in eukaryotes is more complex than a similar process in prokaryotes (*see* above).

118

Elongation of the globin chain

After formation of the complex of globin mRNA and both ribosomal sub-units with bound methionyl-tRNA$_f$ (*see* Fig. 41) the system is able to proceed with the stepwise addition of amino acids from the N-terminal end (*Dintzis*, 1961).

This cycle involves at least three distinct stages (*Lucas-Lenard* and *Lipmann*, 1971): (1) a codon-directed binding of aminoacyl-tRNA to a ribosomal site neighbouring

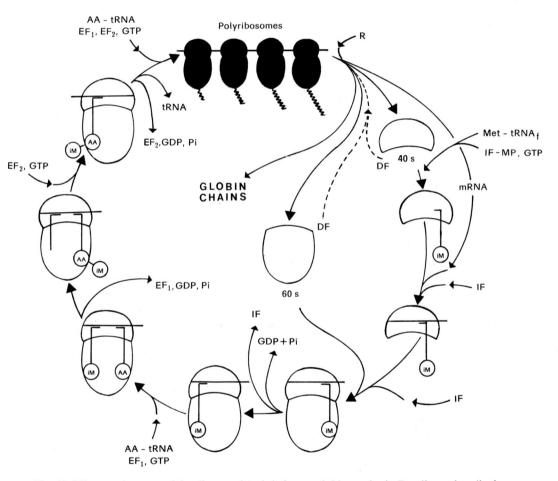

Fig. 42. Ribosomal states and the ribosomal cycle in haemoglobin synthesis. Details are described in the text. 40 s — small ribosomal sub-unit; 60 s — large ribosomal sub-unit; Met-tRNA$_f$ — initiator methionyl-tRNA; AA-tRNA — aminoacyl-tRNA; iM — initiation methionine; IF-MP — homogeneous initiation factor; IF — various initiation factors; EF$_1$, EF$_2$ — elongation factors; R — termination factor; DF — dissociation factor. (Modified from a model originally proposed by *Pestka* (1971) for prokaryotes.)

119

the site occupied by the initiator or peptidyl-tRNA, (2) peptidyl transfer between the newly bound aminoacyl-tRNA and methionyl-tRNA$_f$ or peptidyl tRNA and (3) translocation of both the mRNA and the newly synthesized peptidyl-tRNA from the acceptor (or aminoacyl - A) to the donor (or peptidyl - P) site on the ribosome. After the translocation has taken place, the free acceptor site with the vacant codon binds specifically subsequent aminoacyl-tRNA. At the same time the deacylated tRNA which donated the growing peptide chain (or N-terminal initiation methionine) is released (Fig. 42). The process is repeated continuously; after each translocation reaction site A becomes vacant and a new codon is exposed at the A-site to direct the binding of the next charged tRNA. Then transpeptidation again takes place (*see* 2), i.e. the part of the polypeptide which is formed is transferred to a new amino acid linked to the tRNA at the A-site and the polypeptide chain is prolonged again by one amino acid. The whole ribosome moves thus along the globin mRNA molecule from its 5'-end to the 3'-end till the initiation site at the 5'-end of the message again becomes vacant. Then the whole process of initiation, as described above, is repeated and a further ribosome moves along the messenger. The result is therefore a group of ribosomes on the mRNA, a polyribosome (Fig. 42). On each ribosome a growing chain of different length is attached, depending on its distance from the 5'-end of the mRNA molecule. The metabolic intermediate during globin synthesis on the ribosome is thus peptidyl-tRNA (*Slabough* and *Morris*, 1970).

For the process of elongation in rabbit reticulocytes (and eukaryocytes in general) two protein factors are essential (*Arlinghaus et al.*, 1963, 1964, 1968; *Hardesty et al.*, 1969, 1972). Translocase (EF$_2$ or T$_2$) is required in the translocation reaction (a shift of peptidyl-tRNA from site A to P making site A vacant with simultaneous advance of the ribosome towards the 3'-end of mRNA by one codon); translocase contains or potentiates GTPase activity which is essential for the reaction. The second factor EF$_1$ (T$_1$) is involved in the binding of the amino acyl-tRNA to ribosomes and it cannot be ruled out that it consists of two moieties (*Prather et al.*, 1974). This reaction also requires GTP. During the elongation process, naturally a system catalyzing the peptide bond formation between the carboxyl group of the amino acid residue of the peptide and the amino group of the amino acid which is next in the sequence of the globin chain is essential. In the reaction a structural ribosomal protein, which possesses "transpeptidase" activity and also EF$_1$, GTP and GTP hydrolysis are involved (*Lucas-Lenard* and *Lipmann*, 1971; *Benz* and *Forget*, 1974).

It must be emphasized that special conditions are necessary for the formation of the first peptide bond between the initiating amino acid, methionine, and the N-terminal amino acid of both globin chains, i.e. valine.* *Crystal et al.* (1971) demonstrated that the formation of methionyl-valine dipeptide requires methionyl-tRNA$_f$, initiation

---

*Valine is the N-terminal amino acid of the α- and ß-chain of human and rabbit globin, but not of the human γ-chain.

factor IF-M$_3$ in addition to factors required for methionyl-tRNA$_f$ ribosome binding. Under these conditions the initiation complex can be formed (*see* above) with methionyl-tRNA$_f$ bound in the P-site of this complete initiation complex (*Crystal et al.*, 1971). Moreover, for the formation of the initial dipeptide valyl-tRNA and the elongation factor EF$_1$ are needed. This elongation factor is obviously needed for the binding of valyl-tRNA to site A and then the dipeptide is formed in the above described manner.

Globin chain termination

Under normal circumstances triplets UAG and UAA do not code for any amino acid (*Nirenberg et al.*, 1965). Investigations using mutants of bacteria and later similar investigations with eukaryotes revealed that codons UAA and UAG are terminator codons in both systems. These codons serve as a signal for the release of the completed polypeptide chain which is followed by the release of the ribosome from mRNA.

Investigations on bacterial systems revealed that so-called release factors (R$_1$, R$_2$), which recognize the terminal codons, play a part in the release of the completed chain from the ribosome-mRNA complex. So far it seems that for the recognition of the terminal codon of globin mRNA and release of the globin chain only one R-factor is required (*Goldstein et al.*, 1970; *Beaudet* and *Caskey*, 1971). Binding of the R-factor requires GTP and the release reaction requires GTP hydrolysis; some of the GTPase activity is a property of the R-factor. During the release of the globin chain hydrolysis of the completed globin polypeptide from tRNA seems to involve the R-factor and polypeptidyl transferase (i.e. a peptide bond-forming enzyme). This enzyme forms an integral part of the ribosome and it appears thus that complete globin is released from the ribosome rather than globyl-tRNA. This conclusion is further supported by the fact that it did not prove possible to detect globyl-tRNA in the postmitochondrial supernatant; on the ribosomes, however, completed globyl-tRNA could be found (*Protzel* and *Morris*, 1973).

Rather convincing evidence of the role of the terminal codon as well as of the existence of further nucleotide sequences on globin mRNA beyond the normal terminal codon (*see* p. 103) are two examples from human pathology. Two pathological human haemoglobins with abnormally long α-chains are known; haemoglobin Constant Spring (*Clegg et al.*, 1971b; *Milner et al.*, 1971) and haemoglobin Wayne (*Seid-Akhavan et al.*, 1972). Hb Constant Spring developed by a simple base substitution in the normal termination codon (UAA or UAG). By this substitution the terminal codon changed into a triplet which codes for glutamine (CAA or CAG) and does not serve as a termination signal and thus translation of globin mRNA may proceed further. Hb Wayne developed by a different mechanism which is called frame-shift mutation. By deletion of one base near the end of α-globin mRNA a shift in the mRNA reading frame is caused. This results in an altered sequence of amino acids in the globin chain

121

beyond the site of deletion and in prolongation of the chain. The 142nd triplet which is normally terminal, "lost" its U-base which is read as part of the previous codon coding for the 141st amino acid (C-terminal amino acid of the α-chain) and thus obviously lost its significance as a termination signal. As in the previous case, translation of the globin chain may proceed further.

The model of initiation of globin synthesis (and of proteins in general) assumes the participation of free sub-units. It may thus be expected that the ribosome released from mRNA will dissociate into its sub-units. This dissociation depends on the factor which was isolated from reticulocyte ribosomes (*Davis*, 1971; *Kaempfer* and *Kaufman*, 1972; *Lubsen* and *Davis*, 1972, 1974; *Mizuno* and *Rabinovitz*, 1973; *Merrick et al.*, 1973). It was suggested that the dissociation factor (DF) is identical with IF-M$_3$ (*Kaempfer* and *Kaufman*, 1972) but this view was not confirmed later (*Merrick et al.*, 1973). It appears that two kinds of DF are present in rabbit reticulocytes, one specific for each sub-unit. Every dissociation factor is able to bind with the appropriate sub-unit and stabilizes it against subsequent re-association with the complementary sub-unit (*Lubsen* and *Davis*, 1974).

To sum up, the ribosome after completing one translation round is released from globin mRNA, dissociates into sub-units which enter the pool of free sub-units in the cytoplasm and are ready for the next translation round. This process, along with initiation, growth and termination of globin chain formation is illustrated schematically in Fig. 42.

REGULATION OF GLOBIN SYNTHESIS

Mechanisms of protein synthesis are nowadays relatively well known, starting with genetic information stored in the DNA molecule to transfer of this information into the protein (globin molecule) via specific messenger RNA. These mechanisms were briefly described in the previous sections. In subsequent sections problems of regulation of these processes will be discussed. There exist several levels where regulation of globin synthesis can be implemented. A very appropriate classification was suggested by *Clegg* (1974). Regulation of globin synthesis can take place at the following levels:

(1) Processes taking place at the gene level;
(2) Transcriptional processes including mRNA synthesis, specificity, quantity, timing, etc.;
(3) Post-transcription processes:
   − mRNA processing, transport, stability;
   − chain initiations, elongation, termination and release;
   − protein sub-unit interactions, haem-binding;
   − tetramer formation and stability, etc.

By way of introduction we shall deal very briefly with genetic regulation of globin synthesis. Detailed reviews are available elsewhere (*Ingram*, 1963; *Huehns* and *Shooter*, 1965; *Lehmann* and *Huntsman*, 1974; *Lang* and *Lorkin*, 1976). The number of globin genes varies greatly from one species to the other. For example in man there exist structural genes for ε, α, γ, β and δ-chains whereby α- and γ-genes are duplicated. At present there is sufficient evidence of a close genetic linkage between β-, γ- and δ-chain genetic loci (*Weatherall* and *Clegg*, 1972) but there is no genetic evidence for the linkage of the α-chain loci to non α-chain loci (β, γ, δ).

The homology of structure of β-, γ- and δ-globin chains is of such a type as may be expected for gene products which developed from a common ancestor. *Ingram* (1963) suggested a developmental scheme assuming that β-, γ- and δ-chains may arisen by tandem duplication of a primordial β-like gene. α- and γ-genes probably duplicated quite recently because both α-genes are identical, and there is only one amino acid difference at position 136 between the various γ-genes (*Schroeder et al.*, 1968). These duplications of globin genes are quite common in many animal species but so far their significance is not clear.

The erythroid cell synthesizing haemoglobin is highly specialized and therefore the assumption was made whether amplification and reiteration of specific genes for globin synthesis may not play a part in this specialization. These views were also supported by the finding that some amphibian ribosomal RNA genes undergo reiteration (tandem duplication) or amplification. *Bishop et al.* (1972) and *Bishop* and *Rosbach* (1973) studied the reiteration frequency of duck globin genes by means of hybridization of DNA with mRNA or cDNA and found that only a few copies of globin genes are present in DNA. Similar results were obtained by *Packman et al.* (1972) and *Harrison et al.* (1972). That means that in erythroid cells which form haemoglobin no specific gene amplification exists and the amount of produced globin mRNA is given by the activity of globin DNA template, whereby no pretranscription regulation is involved.

Specific mechanisms controlling transcription of globin genes belong to general problems of expression of specific genes. Elucidation of these mechanisms will resolve one of the basic problems of biology — how to achieve specialization in protein synthesis in differentiated cells when genetic information is ubiquitous. Analysis of views pertaining to gene regulation and transcription processes in the genome of higher organisms are beyond the framework of this monograph and we wish to refer readers interested in these problems to the recent review by *Davidson* and *Britten* (1973). Some problems concerning the regulation of transcription processes, i.e. globin mRNA synthesis are discussed elsewhere (*see* p. 104 and 152).

POST-TRANSCRIPTION CONTROL OF GLOBIN SYNTHESIS

Globin messenger RNA is formed as part of HnRNA which is subject to consider-able metabolic changes. Before this large molecule is processed into mRNA, to the 3'-terminal end of the HnRNA molecule poly(A) sequence is added, probably by the consecutive addition of simple base residues. Most of the HnRNA is turned over in the nucleus. The formed globin pre-mRNA shortens further (at the 5'-terminal end), combines with proteins and is transferred from the nucleus into the cytoplasm as mRNA for globin. At all levels described various regulating factors may play a part, their final goal being to influence the amount of globin mRNA which becomes available in the cytoplasm for translation. Unfortunately none of these events can be recorded by existing methods to assess whether and to what extent regulation mechanisms are involved.

These problems will have to be resolved on nucleated erythroid elements, while so far reticulocytes have mainly been used as an experimental model for investigations of haemoglobin synthesis. The reticulocyte is, on the other hand, a very suitable system for the investigation of the cytoplasmatic control of globin synthesis because it lacks a nucleus. In the interpretation of data obtained from *in vitro* experiments on reticulo-cytes such factors need not be taken into account as e.g. production of mRNA. It must, however, be kept in mind that the reticulocyte is a highly differentiated cell where haemoglobin synthesis gradually declines and all conclusions ensuing from experiments performed on reticulocytes need not necessarily apply to the nucleated erythroblast. There are actually data suggesting that the two types of cells respond in a different way to certain experimental conditions (*Waxman*, 1970).

In subsequent paragraphs we shall discuss two aspects which form part of the post-transcription regulatory processes: the stability of globin mRNA and regulation of translation of mRNA for globin. A more detailed account on the cytoplasmatic level of regulation of haemoglobin synthesis which comprises the control of substrate supply and regulation of haem synthesis in addition to the post-translation fate of globin chains will be presented in a special chapter (p. 135).

Stability of globin mRNA

The life span of individual mRNAs for different chains has not so far been deter-mined, as suitable methods were lacking. Recently, however, very sensitive methods for the detection of minute amounts of mRNA have been elaborated (p. 99) which will probably help to determine the stability of globin mRNA.

There are certain data on relative rates of synthesis of various haemoglobins during maturation of erythroid cells which indirectly indicate the life spans of various RNAs. *Rieder* and *Weatherall* (1965), *Ingram* and *Winslow* (1966) and *Roberts et al.* (1972) found that in reticulocytes haemoglobin A_2 synthesis is completed sooner than syn-thesis of haemoglobin A. It is therefore obvious that the ability to form δ-chains is lost sooner that the ability to form β-chains in cells during reticulocyte maturation. These data, however, provide no information whether mRNA for δ-chains is broken down earlier or whether it cannot be used for protein synthesis. Experimental evidence was also presented indicating that during maturation of the erythroid cell (reticulocyte) γ-chain mRNA declines more rapidly than β-chain mRNA. During incubation of reticulocytes from human umbilical blood earlier arrest of foetal haemoglobin synthesis is apparent (*Prchal* and *Neuwirt*, 1968).

It would certainly be very interesting to investigate the relationship between the life spans of these mRNA for different chains and the length or presence of poly(A) segment which these messengers contain. *Huez et al.* (1974, 1975) and *Marbaix et al,* (1975) provided recently evidence that the poly(A) segment plays an important role in maintaining the stability of globin mRNA; messengers without poly(A) are much less stable.

Del Monte and *Kazazian* (1971) published important results with regard to regulation of mRNA stability in reticulocytes. The authors made use of the well known fact that in reticulocytes incubated with O-methylthreonine α-mRNA contains relatively few ribosomes while in β-mRNA ribosomes are packed to a maximum (*see* Fig. 34). Reticulocytes were incubated for 20 hours with O-methylthreonine and then their ability to form α- and β-chains was investigated. Preincubation of reticulocytes with O-methylthreonine reduced their ability to synthesize α-chains, while the capacity to form β-chains increased considerably, compared with controls. These results indicate that β-mRNA, fully occupied with ribosomes, was in some way protected against inactivation by ribonuclease. These results indicate moreover that life span of mRNA is not *a priori* predetermined.

In this connection it is worth mentioning that the life span of mRNA for some non-haemoglobin proteins is probably shorter that the life span of mRNA for haemoglobin (*Borsook*, 1964; *Edwards*, 1970). The different stability of mRNA for globin and non-haemoglobin proteins was also suggested in mouse primitive yolk sac erythroid cells (*Fantoni et al.*, 1968, *Terada et al.*, 1971). Between gestational days 11 and 13 there is a sharp decrease in the rate of RNA synthesis. Parallel with the drop of RNA synthesis, there is a decrease in the rate of non-globin protein synthesis, whereas globin formation remains unchanged.

Translation control

In the subsequent sections we shall mention factors which control the rate of translation of mRNA. In recent years many important findings were assembled to the control of haemoglobin synthesis at the translation level. In this field, as in other areas of haemoglobin synthesis, views have been gradually developing and some older concepts have already been abandoned. It is obvious that the rate of synthesis of the globin chain depends on the rate of initiation, growth and termination of the chain. Much evidence has been assembled suggesting that the rate of globin synthesis depends on the availability of haem. The possibility can also be considered that the availability of tRNA or globin chains could be factors which control globin formation. Before discussing the question of the level of chain synthesis at which these factors may play a part, the problem of rate limiting steps in globin synthesis must be considered. It is quite evident that the slowest step determines the final rate of chain formation.

Rate limiting step in the synthesis of the globin chain

Dintzis (1961) and later *Naughton* and *Dintzis* (1962) studied the rate and mode of growth of rabbit globin chains. The principle of the method was assessment of radioactivity of the soluble haemoglobin (i.e. haemoglobin released from ribosomes) after pulse-labelling experiments with labelled amino acids for varying periods of time. The radioactive amino acid is incorporated into nascent chains which grow during incubation on the ribosome and after completion they are gradually released. Those chains which were completed first after the beginning of incubation with the radioactive amino acid, contained the label only in a part of the chain near C-terminal amino acid. In the chains completed later, a gradually increasing portion of the polypeptide is labelled, and finally when the incubation lasts sufficiently long, the whole chain up to the N-terminal amino acid is labelled. This period, which gives the time needed for chain formation, was estimated to be 90 seconds. These experiments, as ensues clearly from their principle, revealed that chains are synthesized from the N-terminal in the direction to the C-terminal amino acid, because the labelling gradient in time was reversed. Moreover, it appeared from these first experiments that the growth of the rabbit chain did not take place at a uniform rate. The kinetics of labelling indicated a "slow point" in the α-chain of rabbit globin between the 40th–50th amino acid residue.

Other authors, using a similar experimental technique with human bone marrow, reported non-uniform rates of synthesis of α- as well as β-globin chains with a break point around position 90. *Winslow* and *Ingram* (1966) and *Ingram* and *Winslow* (1966) postulated at this site a control point of globin chain synthesis and explained the slowing by the addition of the prosthetic haem group.

Hunt et al. (1968a), however, raised serious objections against the original method where the rate of translation of different areas of mRNA was assessed by measuring the radioactivity of soluble globin. These authors used a more direct method and assessed the specific activity of peptides obtained from nascent chains growing on polyribosomes of rabbit reticulocytes incubated with leucine-^{3}H. When the specific activities of peptides were plotted against their position in the protein, they were on a straight line. These authors thus did not find any evidence supporting the original assumption that ribosomes move at a different rate along the mRNA. In other words, there was no evidence of any rate limiting area during chain growth. In subsequent research *Hunt, Hunter* and *Munro* (1969b) ruled out the possibility that termination of globin chain formation may be the slowest step of peptide formation. Control at this level (i.e. the terminal stage) was originally assumed by *Colombo* and *Baglioni* (1966) and *Baglioni* and *Campana* (1967).

Similarly *Luppis et al.* (1970) were unable to prove a rate limiting area during growth or release of chains of rabbit globin. In keeping with these investigations *Clegg et al.* (1968) and *Rieder* (1972) did not find any evidence suporting the view that there exists a control point which divides areas with a different rate of human globin formation.

More recent experiments are thus strongly in favour of the idea that the control of globin chain synthesis takes place rather at the level of initiation than during elongation or termination of the chain. For this reason the original concept of *Itano* (1965) that the limited availability of certain tRNA molecules could delay elongation and thus determine the rate of the entire translation is rather unlikely. Nevertheless attention must be drawn to the fact that some authors still consider the possibility of a regulating role of tRNA availability during translation of globin mRNA (*Smith*, 1975). tRNA availability as a controlling factor in globin synthesis in erythroid cells could actually participate in certain pathological conditions. It may be assumed that a certain codon could change by mutation into a triplet which codes for the same amino acid (this is possible because of degeneration of the code) but requires a different tRNA which is present in the cell in limited amounts.

Synchronization of synthesis of different chains

The coordination of synthesis of the two main globin chains, α and β, has been the subject of considerable interest. Rates of chain synthesis are very subtly coordinated and thus only a small excess of free α-chains is present in the cytoplasm (*Heywood et al.*, 1966; *Shaeffer*, 1967). Similarly there also exists a very small amount of the αβ-dimer which is an intermediary product in haemoglobin synthesis (*Heywood*, 1967; *Tavill et al.*, 1968; *Heywood* and *Finch*, 1970). Cumulation of the αβ-dimer during haemoglobin synthesis is prevented by the dependence of chain formation on availability of haem and by the immediate combination of the dimer with *de novo* produced haem. Based on investigation in cell-free systems it seems that synthesis of α- and β-chains is controlled by feedback mechanisms whereby a central role is ascribed to α-chains. Addition of α-chains to cell-free systems from rabbit reticulocytes inhibits the synthesis of α-chains but not that of β-chains (*Blum* and *Schapira*, 1967; *Blum et al.*, 1969, 1970, 1972; *Shaeffer et al.*, 1969); if the free α-chain pool is first removed from the system, α-chains even stimulate the synthesis of β-chains (*Blum et al.*, 1969, 1970). β-chains inhibit in similar cell-free systems their own synthesis (*Blum* and *Schapira*, 1967; *Blum et al.*, 1969, 1970, 1972; *Shaeffer et al.*, 1967, 1969). It is possible that this effect of β-chains is not direct. Added β-chains combine with α-chains and as a result of depletion of the free α-chain pool the release of β-chains from polyribosomes is reduced (*Shaeffer et al.*, 1967, 1969).

Investigations on intact cells agree only partly with these results in cell-free systems. In intact cells it is possible to inhibit selectively the synthesis of one globin chain, if this chain contains isoleucine, by addition of an isoleucine isostere, O-methyl-1-threonine (OMT) (*Honig*, 1967; *Kazazian* and *Freedman*, 1968; *Rabinovitz et al.*, 1969). In human haemoglobin the synthesis of the γ-chain which forms part of haemoglobin F can be selectively inhibited by OMT. Under these circumstances, however, the synthesis of the α-chain proceeds at the normal rate and the free α-chains accumulate in cells (*Honig et al.*, 1969). This result provides evidence against the regulation of α-chain synthesis in intact cells by a mechanism of feedback inhibition. Another suitable model for similar investigations are reticulocytes of some rabbits the β-chains of which do not contain isoleucine, while the α-chains do. As may be expected, incubation of reticulocytes from such rabbits with OMT is associated with inhibition of α-chain formation. OMT, however, did not inhibit β-chain synthesis (*Rabinovitz et al.*, 1969; *Wolf et al.*, 1973; *Garrick et al.*, 1975) and in experiments of *Rabinovitz* and *Garrick* synthesis of β-chains was even stimulated. Rabbit reticulocytes, however, contain a pool of free α-chains (*see* above) which need not be completely exhausted by incubation with OMT. Therefore a similar experiment was performed with bone marrow (*Wolf et al.*, 1973), which does not contain free α-chains. Inhibition of α-chain synthesis by OMT was associated under these conditions by a significantly reduced rate of β-chain synthesis. These results indicate thus that also in intact erythroid cells coordinated synthesis of α- and β-globin chains can at least partly be the result of the modifying action of α-chains on β-chain synthesis.

It is, however, obvious that even if there is a certain feedback regulation of globin chain synthesis in erythroid cells, this mechanism is relatively ineffective in severe disorders of chain synthesis, such as in thalassaemia. In α-thalassaemia − where the synthesis of the α-chain is reduced, in the cytoplasm tetramers of the β-chains are present (*Bank* and *Marks*, 1969). Similarly in β-thalassaemia − where the synthesis of β-chains is reduced − synthesis of α-chains proceeds at the normal rate and this results in accumulation of the α-chains in the cytoplasm (*Fessas* and *Loukopoulos*, 1964; *Bank et al.*, 1968).

Coordination of α- and β-globin chain synthesis also depends, no doubt, on relative amounts of mRNA for both main chains and on relative translation rates of these mRNA molecules. In the rabbit (*Hunt, Hunter* and *Munro*, 1968, 1969a,b) and human (*Clegg et al.*, 1971a; *Nathan et al.*, 1971) reticulocytes α-chains are formed on small polyribosomes while β-chains are synthesized on larger polyribosomes. Since the translation rate of α- and β-globin mRNA seems to be equal (*Lodish* and *Jacobsen*, 1972), the initiation of mRNA translation for β-chains is more rapid than the initiation of translation of the α-chain (*Nathan et al.*, 1971). The more rapid initiation of the β-chain would imply, however, a greater production of β-globin chains and it may therefore be assumed that the cell contains more mRNA for α-chains than for β-chains (*Lodish*, 1971) in order to maintain the equilibrium in the formation of

128

the two main globin chains. This assumption was later confirmed by direct assay of α- and β-polyribosomes by means of immunoprecipitation techniques (*Boyer et al.*, 1974).

It is thus obvious that coordination of the production of the two main haemoglobin chains is a very complicated process which cannot be explained merely by feedback inhibition of chain formation at the cytoplasmatic level. During balanced chain synthesis the number of mRNA molecules for α- and β-chains as well as different rates of chain initiation play a part. So far it is impossible to elaborate a complete pattern of the mechanisms which determine the different mRNA content in cytoplasm and differences in initiation rate. It may be, however, assumed that these mechanisms are subjected to some feedback control.

The role of haem in globin synthesis

Kruh and *Borsook* (1956) were the first who suggested that the rates of haem and globin synthesis are coordinated. After 1964 it became apparent that the basis of this coordination is the dependence of globin synthesis on the availability of haem (*Bruns* and *London*, 1965; *London et al.*, 1964; *Waxman* and *Rabinovitz*, 1965; *Rabinovitz* and *Waxman*, 1965; *Neuwirt et al.*, 1968; *Schulman*, 1968; *Poňka et al.*, 1970).

The dependence of globin synthesis on availability of haem in intact reticulocytes was revealed conclusively by experiments with depletion of intracellular haem induced by various inhibitors. The incubation of reticulocytes under conditions of iron deficiency or with iron chelates (*Waxman* and *Rabinovitz*, 1965, 1966; *Grayzel et al.*, 1966; *Rabinovitz* and *Waxman*, 1965) and with other inhibitors of haem synthesis such as isoniazide (INH) (*Poňka et al.*, 1970; *Fuhr* and *Gengozian*, 1973; *Neuwirt et al.*, 1975b), lead (*Waxman* and *Rabinovitz*, 1966; *White* and *Harvey*, 1972; *White* and *Hoffbrand* 1974), ethanol (*Feedman et al.*, 1975) or benzene (*Forte et al.*, 1976) is associated with inhibition of globin formation. Globin synthesis, inhibited as a result of primary inhibition of haem synthesis, can be restored by addition of haemin to the incubation system. The reparation of globin synthesis, inhibited by isoniazide (INH), by addition of haemin to reticulocytes may serve as an example (*Poňka et al.*, 1970) (Table 13). Moreover, it is possible to restore globin synthesis, inhibited by isoniazide, by addition of δ-aminolaevulinic acid (*see* p. 78) which regenerates the endogenous haem pool in reticulocytes (*Neuwirt et al.*, 1975b). Similarly, in patients with sideroblastic anaemia, where haem synthesis is primarily inhibited (*see* p. 168), globin synthesis is inhibited and the amount of the αβ-dimer rises in erythroid cells (*White et al.*, 1971). Addition of haemin to such erythroid cells stimulates synthesis of the α-as well as β-chain and eliminates the pool of free αβ-dimer (*see also* p. 140).

Despite the immense effort to explain the mechanism of the action of haem on globin synthesis, this problem has not been satisfactorily resolved. Early experiments had already revealed that reticulocyte incubation with iron chelates is associated with disaggregation of polyribosomes to free ribosomes. This disaggregation can

Table 13

60-minute incorporation of glycine-2-^{14}C into haem and globin and of leucine-^{14}C into globin of control reticulocytes and of reticulocytes incubated with INH or haemin

	Incorporation of				
	Glycine-2-^{14}C into			Leucine-^{14}C into	
	Haem (cpm/mg)	Globin (cpm/mg)	% of appropriate control	Globin (cpm/mg)	% of appropriate control
Control	1,598	69	100.0	171	100.0
Haemin (10^{-4}M)	1,090	97	140.6	296	173.1
INH (10^{-2}M)	132	25	100.0	44	100.0
INH (10^{-2}M) + haemin (10^{-4}M) (haemin added in the same time as INH)	132	116	464.0	376	854.5
INH (10^{-2}M) + haemin (10^{-4}M) (haemin added 30 minutes after INH)	133	133	532.0	403	915.5

Cells were preincubated with or without INH 40 minutes before addition of the label. Cells in the last group were preincubated for 30 minutes with INH only, then haemin and after 10 minutes isotope were added (i.e. at the same time as to all other samples). Each value represents the mean of four samples. (From *Poňka et al.*, 1970. Reproduced with the permission of the Academic Press, Inc., New York.)

be prevented by addition of haemin to the incubation mixture (*Grayzel et al.*, 1966; *Waxman* and *Rabinovitz*, 1966). *Rabinovitz et al.* (1969) assumed later that the stabilizing action of haem on polyribosomes rules out the role of haem in terminal stages of globin synthesis. Originally it was suggested that haem is involved at this level of formation of the globin molecule. If haem facilitated the completion of globin chain synthesis, we could expect disaggregation of ribosomes after addition of exogenous haemin to reticulocytes. There is also evidence that haemin does not join nascent polypeptide chains on ribosomes (*Felicetti et al.*, 1968; *Waxman et al.*, 1967; *Morris* and *Liang*, 1968). From these data ensues that haem probably controls globin synthesis at the level of peptide chain initiation.

To resolve the question of whether and how haem acts at the initiation level, cell-free systems from reticulocytes were used. In this connection it must be emphasized that in the cell-free system from reticulocytes haem is quite indispensible for the maintenance of globin synthesis. In rabbit reticulocyte lysate very rapidly the ability of initiation of new globin chains is lost (*Schweet et al.*, 1958; *Lamform* and *Knopf*,

1964). After addition of haemin to this lysate at the onset of incubation the capacity is established to initiate new rounds of globin synthesis and thus the capacity of the system to synthesize protein is prolonged from ca 5 minutes to 15–20 minutes (*Zucker* and *Schulman*, 1967, 1968; *Adamson et al.*, 1968, 1969a,b; *Maxwell* and *Rabinovitz*, 1969; *Howard et al.*, 1970b; *Gross* and *Rabinovitz*, 1972a,b). The later haemin is added after onset of incubation of the lysate, the smaller is its effect till eventually by about the 15th minute the added haem is no longer effective in stimulating protein synthesis (*Adamson et al.*, 1969a, 1972; *Gross* and *Rabinovitz*, 1972a, 1973; *Maxwell et al.*, 1971; *Hunt et al.*, 1972).

Rabinovitz et al. demonstrated that haem deficiency in the cell-free system is associated with the formation of an inhibitor of protein synthesis. When the post-ribosomal supernatant from reticulocytes is incubated at temperatures above 37°C in the absence of haemin, an inhibitor of polypeptide chain initiation is formed. This inhibitor which is denoted as haemin-controlled repressor (HCR) is formed from a precursor of HCR (prorepressor, proinhibitor) (*Maxwell* and *Rabinovitz*, 1969; *Howard et al.*, 1970b; *Maxwell et al.*, 1971; *Gross* and *Rabinovitz*, 1972a,b, 1973; *Legon et al.*, 1973). HCR formed within the first 30 minutes can be inactivated by haemin (*Gross* and *Rabinovitz*, 1972b) and therefore was named "reversible inhibitor". The inhibitor is a protein with a molecular weight of $4 \pm 1 \times 10^5$ daltons (*Adamson et al.*, 1972; *Mizuno et al.*, 1972; *Gross* and *Rabinovitz*, 1972a). After a prolonged incubation period of the reticulocyte lysate an "irreversible inhibitor" accumulates which is not affected by haemin (*Gross* and *Rabinovitz*, 1972a,b; *Maxwell* and *Rabinovitz*, 1969; *Maxwell et al.*, 1971; *Gross*, 1974a):

$$\text{proinhibitor-haemin} \rightleftarrows \text{proinhibitor} \rightleftarrows \text{reversible} \rightarrow \text{irreversible}$$

proinhibitor-haemin ⇌ proinhibitor ⇌ reversible → irreversible
complex   +   inhibitor   inhibitor
                 haemin
                   +
              globin → methaemoglobin

The proinhibitor also gives rise to another molecule termed "intermediate inhibitor". The intermediate form is not directly inactivated by haemin but is inactivated in systems where protein synthesis takes place (*Gross*, 1974b). The majority of investigations so far were conducted with the irreversible inhibitor; it must, however, be kept in mind that the irreversible inhibitor can hardly participate as a physiological regulating factor which maintains the equilibrium between the rates of haem and globin synthesis. It is, however, possible that the reversible inhibitor has the same mechanism of action as the irreversible form.

HCR causes disaggregation of polyribosomes under conditions of protein synthesis. The block which the inhibitor causes in polypeptide chain initiation may be overcome by a factor partially purified from a high salt wash of reticulocyte ribosomes (i.e. containing IF) (*Adamson et al.*, 1972; *Mizuno et al.*, 1972; *Kaempfer* and

Kaufman, 1972; *Beuzard* and *London*, 1974; *Clemens et al.*, 1974, 1975) or by a factor found in the postribosomal supernatant fraction (*Gross*, 1975). The activity of the inhibitor can be markedly reduced by cyclic AMP (*Legon et al.*, 1974; *Levin et al.*, 1975; *Ernst et al.*, 1976). GTP blocks the formation of this inhibitor, while ATP was found to stimulate this process (*Balkow et al.*, 1975). Regardless of whether these factors play a part in intact erythroid cells under physiological conditions or not, it is obvious that haemin is not the only, i.e. specific factor which interferes with the metabolism of the inhibitor.

As has already been mentioned, the inhibitor acts at the level of initiation and evidence was provided that HCR prevents the association of methionyl-tRNA$_f$ with the small ribosomal sub-unit (*Legon et al.*, 1973; *Balkow et al.*, 1973a). It is, however, also possible that HCR promotes deacylation of methionyl-tRNA occurring after initiator tRNA binding to the 40s sub-unit (*Balkow et al.*, 1973b). From the previous text ensued (*see* p. 115) that for the initiation of globin formation also formyl methionyl-tRNA may be used; in that case the system derived from reticulocytes is unable to cleave formyl methionine. It is therefore interesting that the initiation of globin synthesis by formylmethionyl-tRNA is not inhibited under conditions when the presence of HCR can be expected in the reticulocyte lysate (*Cahn* and *Lubin*, 1975). HCR thus evidently acts at the step of natural initiation.

All above-mentioned results with cell-free systems indicate that haem controls a step in the initiation process before the involvement of mRNA. This suggests that the control of protein synthesis by haem should not be specific for globin. Therefore it is not surprising that HCR inhibits the synthesis of non-haemoglobin proteins (*Mizuno et al.*, 1972) and that haemin stimulates translation of non-globin proteins in reticulocyte lysate (*Mathews et al.*, 1973; *Beuzard et al.*, 1973; *Lodish* and *Desalu*, 1973). Similarly in intact reticulocytes with an experimentally induced haem deficiency the synthesis of non-globin proteins declines and can be raised by an increase in the level of the intracellular haem pool (*Neuwirt et al.*, 1975b).

In connection with these results, which clearly indicate the non-specific character of the action of haem, the question arises why in some systems haem interferes with the synthesis of only one chain. For example haemin was shown to stimulate α- but not β-globin synthesis in *Xenopus* oocytes injected with rabbit globin mRNA (*Giglioni et al.*, 1973). Similarly, in human erythroid cells with haem deficiency inhibition of α-chain synthesis predominates (*White* and *Hoffbrand*, 1974). On the other hand, the rate of globin mRNA translation in non-reticulocyte cell-free systems is practically not influenced by addition of haemin (*Mathews*, 1972; *Mathews et al.*, 1972; *Borová et al.*, 1976).

Thus doubts arise whether the results obtained in cell-free systems can be applied to the control of globin synthesis in intact erythroid cells. As was emphasized in the introduction of this section, one fact is beyond doubt: primary inhibition of haem synthesis in intact erythroid cells is associated with inhibition of globin synthesis.

132

Addition of haem can restore the inhibited globin synthesis (e.g. *Grayzel et al.*, 1966; *Waxman* and *Rabinovitz*, 1966; *Poňka et al.*, 1970; *Fuhr* and *Gengozian*, 1973; *White et al.*, 1971; *White* and *Hoffbrand*, 1974; *Neuwirt et al.*, 1975b). It is, however, not clear by what mechanism haem acts on globin synthesis in these intact cells. So far evidence has not been provided that an inhibitor similar to HCR is formed in reticulocytes incubated e.g. with isoniazide (INH).* Moreover, there is a remarkable difference in the responsiveness to haemin between the protein synthesis in intact reticulocytes incubated in the absence of endogenous haem synthesis (*Poňka et al.*, 1970; *Fuhr* and *Gengozian*, 1973; *Neuwirt et al.*, 1975b) and that in the reticulocyte lysate preincubated without added haemin. In the intact rabbit reticulocyte with inhibited haem synthesis for 60–90 minutes haem is still capable to restore globin synthesis (Table 13; *see* also *Neuwirt et al.*, 1975b). However, addition of haemin to the reticulocyte lysate about 15 minutes after the beginning of incubation is rarely effective in increasing protein synthesis in this system (*Adamson et al.*, 1969a, 1972; *Howard et al.*, 1970; *Hunt et al.*, 1972). The controversial point is thus that in the lysate the irreversible form of HCR would be formed certainly after 60–90 minutes. On the other hand, in intact reticulocytes incubated with INH either the reversible or intermediate form of the inhibitor is formed, or globin synthesis inhibition is perhaps caused by a different mechanism.

Evidence that an inhibitor might be involved in the haem-mediated control of globin synthesis in intact reticulocytes was recently presented by *Schulman* (1975) and *Hunter* and *Jackson* (1975). Both papers are motivated by the observation previously described that at low temperatures (about 25°C) the translation repressor is not formed in reticulocyte lysate incubated without haem. *Schulman* observed that intact reticulocytes incubated for prolonged periods in the absence of iron (haem deficiency is induced) at a temperature of 25°C preserve their ability to respond to the addition of iron by increased globin synthesis. On the other hand, in cells incubated under identical conditions at 35°C globin synthesis cannot be stimulated later by addition of iron. Moreover, reticulocyte incubation at temperatures of about 25°C, when haem synthesis is markedly inhibited, leads to cumulation of the globin dimer in cells. In other words at these low temperatures (25°C) globin synthesis can take place relatively more rapidly and thus independently of haem synthesis.

Hunter and *Jackson* (1975) incubated reticulocytes at various temperatures and observed that at temperatures below 30°C incubation in the presence of dipyridyl (an iron chelate) did not cause inhibition of protein synthesis. At temperatures be-

---

* However, recent results of *Freedman* and *Rosman* (1976) seem to indicate that HCR forms in haem-deficient intact erythroid cells and that its appearance may be responsible for the inhibition of globin synthesis. These investigators isolated and partially purified the translational repressor from intact rabbit reticulocytes incubated *in vitro* with either dipyridyl (an iron chelating agent) or with ethanol. Both agents decrase the rate of haem formation and inhibit protein synthesis in intact reticulocytes.

tween 30°C–40°C dipyridyl does not inhibit globin synthesis during the first minutes of incubation. Later, however, a period of gradual decline in the rate of incorporation follows which gives rise to a second phase when reticulocytes adopt a slow linear rate of protein synthesis. If cells from the second phase are shifted to a lower temperature, a burst of protein synthesis occurs. These results seem to indicate that in the presence of dipyridyl globin synthesis declines due to the inhibitor which is formed at temperatures above 25°C.

As far as the mechanism of action of haem in globin synthesis is concerned, many questions remain open, as ensues from the previous text. HCR is not a specific factor interfering with globin synthesis (*see* above) and moreover its effect can be mimicked by many other substances such as double-stranded RNA (*Ehrenfeld* and *Hunt*, 1971; *Darnbrough et al.*, 1972; *Clemens et al.*, 1975) and oxidized glutathione (*Kosower et al.*, 1971, 1972; *Clemens et al.*, 1975). Conclusive evidence is also lacking that HCR is formed in intact reticulocytes with haem deficiency and that it thus inhibits globin synthesis in this way.* It is therefore possible that a factor more important for the coordination of the two synthetic processes is the involvement of haem in normal haemoglobin assembly from globin (*see* p. 140). Haem reduces the size of the pool of α-chains and αβ-dimers and thus renders more rapid chain formation possible by reducing feedback inhibition exerted by free globin chains (*see* p. 127).

Note added in proof:
Recent reports have suggested that HCR may act as a specific protein kinase, phosphorylating a 38 000 molecular weight sub-unit of an initiation factor that promotes binding of the initiator tRNA to the 40 s sub-unit [*Levin D. H., Ranu R. S., Ernst V., London I. M.* (1976): Proc. nat. Acad. Sci. (Wash.) *73*, 3112; *Kramer G., Cimadevilla J. M., Hardesty B.* (1976): Proc. nat. Acad. Sci. (Wash.): *73*, 3078]. The prorepressor, which has little inhibitory activity, has little capacity to phosphorylate the 38 000 molecular weight component of this initiation factor. Prolonged warming of the prorepressor produces the translational inhibitor and protein kinase that phosphorylates the 38 000 molecular weight sub-unit. Haemin prevents the formation of both the inhibitory and protein kinase activities [*Gross M., Mendelewski J.* (1977): Biochem. biophys. Res. Commun. *74*, 559].

* See footnote on page 133.

5. REGULATION OF HAEMOGLOBIN SYNTHESIS

COORDINATION OF HAEM AND GLOBIN SYNTHESES

The haemoglobin molecule contains two different globin chains and haem. These three components are synthesized in all erythroid cells in equivalent amounts. It seems that this coordination of the equivalent haem and globin chain production takes place in the cytoplasm and is not under genetic control because haem and globin syntheses are also coordinated in reticulocytes where no DNA and RNA are formed.

The erythroid cell may be compared with a factory where one machine, polyribosomes, produces two globin chains and another machine, mitochondria, produces haem. Although haem as well as globin are produced at two different sites, the control of their formation is extremely effective. Diminished globin or haem synthesis is associated almost immediately or after only a very small delay with restricted synthesis of the other component.

It appears that coordinated haemoglobin synthesis and its regulation is implemented only by the control of *de novo* synthesis of haem or globin. Evidence was found in several tissues that haem is broken down in the endoplasmatic reticulum by the enzyme haem oxygenase. So far it is not known whether haem oxygenase is also effective in erythroid cells and whether it participates in the regulation of haemoglobin synthesis. That during intensive haemoglobin synthesis in erythroid cells all haem transported to the microsomes combines with the globin chains and that the situation practically never develops when it is broken down by haem oxygenase cannot be ruled out. Recent data, however (*Yannoni* and *Robinson*, 1975; *Glass et al.*, 1975b) indicate that not only liver but also erythroid cells contain a haem-destroying system. This conclusion follows from the observation that in both cell types there is a haem pool (with a very rapid turnover). Some reports indicate that in thalassaemia an excess of globin chains can be broken down by proteolytic enzymes (*Bank* and *O'Donnel*, 1969). So far in normal erythroid cells, however, proteolytic breakdown of globin chains has not been demonstrated, although this possibility must be taken into consideration.

REGULATORY ROLE OF HAEM

It is assumed that haem may belong to the group of low molecular substances with general regulatory properties. Haem inhibits its own synthesis in erythroid cells (*Karibian* and *London*, 1965), most probably by its inhibitory action on iron release from transferrin (*Poňka* and *Neuwirt*, 1969, 1974; *Poňka et al.*, 1974). The presence of haem is also indispensable for globin synthesis (*Bruns* and *London*, 1965; *Zucker* and *Schulman*, 1968; *Poňka et al.*, 1970). In some way haem affects the initiation of globin chains (*see* p. 131). It is of interest that haem not only affects globin synthesis but also stimulates the synthesis of some other proteins (*Beuzard et al.*, 1973). Haem also inhibits glycine transport into rabbit erythroid cells (*Neuwirt* and *Poňka*, 1972). Experiments in Granick's laboratory provided conclusive evidence that in cultures of chick-embryo livers haem inhibits ALA synthetase formation at the translation level (*Sassa* and *Granick*, 1971). Haem in reticulocytes inhibits DNA polymerase and RNA-dependent RNA polymerase (*Byrnes et al.*, 1974; *Downey et al.*, 1973).

If haem is to combine with globin chains near polyribosomes, it must be transported there from mitochondria. So far it is not clear whether during this extramitochondrial transport haem is transferred free or as part of some complex (*Israels et al.*, 1975). Similarly the question of the relative affinity of haem to various intracellular proteins has not been completely elucidated. It seems that various proteins can accelerate or retard the intracellular mobility of haem (*Poňka et al.*, 1973b) and that the transport of haem from mitochondria to microsomes is mediated by different carriers. The great affinity of globin chains for haem can obviously release haem from the bond with the carrier. According to *Israel's* concept haem which has not yet combined with the apoprotein should be denoted as uncommitted haem.

Table 14

Scheme of the experimental procedure used for the separation of free haem and of haem bound to non-haemoglobin proteins

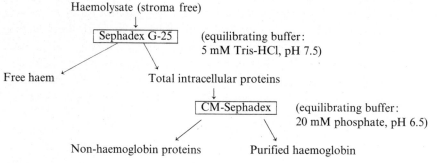

(From *Neuwirt et al.*, 1972. Reproduced with the permission of Elsevier/North-Holland Biomedical Press B.V., Amsterdam.)

All above controversial points regarding the role and presence of haem stimulated experiments to detect in what form haem is present in cells.

Reticulocytes were incubated with radioiron of a high specific activity, bound to transferrin. The haemolysate from these cells was passed through a Sephadex G 25 column. Free labelled haem is retained in the column but can subsequently be eluted by means of an eluting solution containing 3% serum albumin. Labelled haem bound to non-haemoglobin proteins was isolated by separation of non-haemoglobin protein by chromatography on CM Sephadex (*see* Table 14). About 96% of the radioactivity of non-haemoglobin haem is bound to protein and only about 4% of labelled haem seems to be in a free form (*Neuwirt et al.*, 1972).

The content of free haem in the haemolysate of reticulocytes incubated with INH is very low, obviously because INH inhibits haem synthesis. On the other hand, the

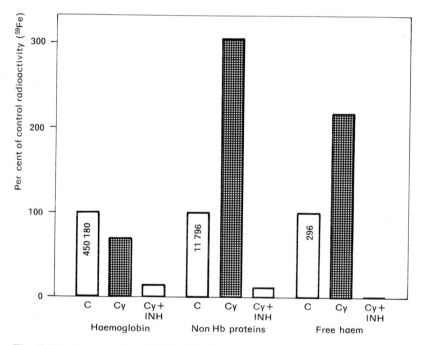

Fig. 43. The incorporation of ^{59}Fe into various haem pools of reticulocytes incubated with specific inhibitors of globin and haem synthesis. The cells were incubated for 60 min at 37°C. ^{59}Fe bound to transferrin of plasma was added after 5 min preincubation with the inhibitors. 1.80 ml of stroma-free haemolysate (corresponding to 0.780 ml of packed red cells) were applied to the column of Sephadex G-25 and in the aliquot of protein eluate haemoglobin from non-haemoglobin proteins was separated (*see Neuwirt et al.*, 1972). The amount of non-haemoglobin proteins (determined at 280 nm, the calibration curve with the human serum albumin) was approx. 10% of all intracellular proteins. Values presented in columns give the radioactivities of appropriate controls. C – control; Cy – cycloheximide. For details *see Neuwirt et al.* (1972).

free haem content is substantially raised in reticulocytes with inhibited protein synthesis (Fig. 43). In reticulocytes with inhibited globin formation a considerable amount of non-haemoglobin haem accumulates also in mitochondria (*Poňka et al.,* 1973).

Further evidence that the radioactivity found in non-haemoglobin haem is actually radioactivity of haem synthesized *de novo* in reticulocytes was provided by experiments where reticulocytes were incubated with glycine-2-^{14}C and where the results were the same as during incubation with [59]Fe (Fig. 44).

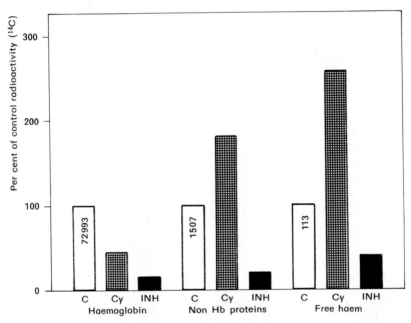

Fig. 44. The incorporation of glycine -2-^{14}C into various haem pools of reticulocytes incubated with specific inhibitors of globin and haem synthesis. The cells were incubated for 60 min at 37°C. Glycine-2-^{14}C was added after 5 min of preincubation with inhibitors. 1.80 ml of stroma-free haemolysate (corresponding to 0.794 ml of packed red cells) were applied to the column of Sephadex G-25 and in the aliquot of protein eluate haemoglobin was separated from non-haemoglobin proteins (*see Neuwirt et al.,* 1972). Values presented in columns give the radioactivities of appropriate controls. C — control; Cy — cycloheximide. For details *see Neuwirt et al.* (1972).

So far it is very difficult to assess the actual amount of free and bound haem in reticulocytes. The concentration of free haem, which has been estimated only very roughly, seems to be of the order of 10^{-6}M in reticulocytes (*Neuwirt et al.,* 1972). *Glass et al.* (1975b) recently reported that reticulocytes as well as less mature nucleated red-cell precursors contained a pool of preformed non-haemoglobin haem. It was

138

suggested, on the basis of indirect evidence, that nucleated erythroid elements contain a larger haem pool than reticulocytes.

Bunn and *Jandl* (1968) found evidence that haemoglobin oxidation increases the dissociation of haem from haemoglobin and concluded that the regulatory role of haem could be effected by haem formed from oxidized haemoglobin. Newly synthesized globin in reticulocytes contains oxidized haem groups (*Schulman et al.*, 1974) and it seems that haem from ferrihaemoglobin may be incorporated in newly formed globin. *Schulman et al.* actually showed that addition of ferrihaemoglobin to reticulocytes and to the cell-free system of these cells in both instances significantly stimulated globin synthesis. It was revealed that globin dimers which are intermediates in haemoglobin synthesis form tetramers in the presence of ferrihaemoglobin. It has long been known that haem after combination with dimers renders the formation of tetramers possible. *Schulman* and co-workers were also able to prove that the action of ferrihaemoglobin can be ascribed to released haem. *Schulman* made the assumption that the small ferrihaemoglobin pool in maturing erythroid cells is in equilibrium with haem synthesized by mitochondria and with haem present in microsomes at the site of globin synthesis. The existence, therefore, of some specific intracellular haem carrier which takes haem from mitochondria to microsomes need not necessarily be assumed. The results obtained in our laboratory, however, suggest that the decisive factor in the formation of the so-called uncommitted haem is the relation between the rate of haem and globin syntheses rather than the level of ferrihaemoglobin.

MUTUAL RELATIONS BETWEEN HAEM AND GLOBIN SYNTHESES

The basic principle of the regulation of haemoglobin synthesis is the dependence of globin synthesis on the presence of haem and the feedback inhibition of haem synthesis by haem. Addition of haemin to reticulocytes stimulates the synthesis of α- and β-chains and increases haemoglobin production. The effect of haemin on globin chain initiation is discussed on p. 131. *Tavill et al.* (1968, 1972) elaborated, based on their experiments with haem, a model of the control of haemoglobin synthesis (Fig. 45).

This model assumes that the synthesis of α-chains is greater than the synthesis of β-chains. Completed β-chains released from polyribosomes combine immediately with newly released α-chains and form with them $\alpha\beta$-dimers (1). An excess of α-chains creates a pool of α-chains (2). β-chains combine either with α-chains from the pool or with newly formed α-chains just released from polyribosomes. In case of haem deficiency a pool of the $\alpha\beta$-dimer is formed because haem is needed for conversion of the $\alpha\beta$-dimer to the haemoglobin tetramer (4). It is assumed that haem coordinates the assembly of the α- and β-chains by facilitating their mutual combination after release of both chains from polyribosomes. In the presence of haem the α-chains do not enter the pool of free α-chains. In summary, haem is required for normal haemoglobin assembly from αβ-dimer. If there is a state of haem deficiency, there is accumulation of αβ-dimers which probably inhibit globin chain termination and release from polyribosomes.

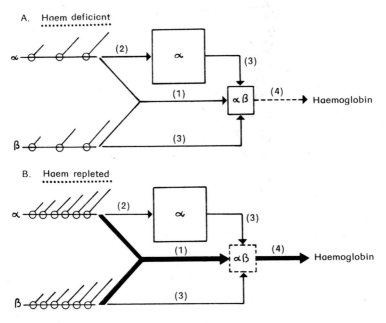

Fig. 45. A proposed model of haemoglobin biosynthesis. The diagram illustrates the effects of added haemin. (a) enhanced polyribosome formation and synthesis of both α- and ß-chains, (b) promotion of the assembly of newly synthesized α- and ß-chains (pathway 1), and (c) conversion of αβ dimers to haemoglobin tetramers with elimination of an αβ-pool (pathway 4). In spite of these effects, excess α-chain synthesis is maintained (pathway 2), the α-chain pool persists and continues to be labelled, and α-chains from the pool continue to combine with newly synthesized ß-chains (pathway 3) so that although the α : ß ratio rises it does not reach 1. (From *Tavill et al.*, 1968. Reproduced with the permission of the authors and the American Society of Biological Chemists, Inc., Bethesda.)

It seems that in the course of reticulocyte maturation globin synthesis persists longer than haem synthesis (*Schulman*, 1968). Therefore free globin should be detectable in erythrocytes. The presence of free globin in red cells was actually demonstrated (*Winterhalter* and *Huehns*, 1963). *Winterhalter et al.* (1969) identified free globin in the haemolysate of normal red cells by means of haemin-^{59}Fe which combines with this free globin. This method is based on the observation that globin can be separated from haemoglobin A by means of column chromatography (*Winterhalter* and *Huehns*, 1964) and that haem reacts with globin and haemoglobin

140

is formed. Using this method it was found that a small fraction of the cellular proteins combines with the added haemin to form a substance which has the spectral, chromatografic and electrophoretic properties of haemoglobin A. This fraction accounts for roughly 0.2% of haemoglobin A isolated from the haemolysate.

This free globin is probably a mixture of the αβ-dimer and $\alpha_2\beta_2$-tetramer partly saturated with haem. Experiments *in vitro* to investigate haemoglobin synthesis revealed that free globin is a precursor in the formation of haemoglobin in nucleated erythroid cells, while in mature erythrocytes it is the residue of excessive globin production (*Heywood* and *Finch*, 1970). This last statement is supported by the finding that an equal amount of free globin is found in reticulocytes and mature red cells.

The percentage of free globin is constant. Isolated globin is, however, very unstable in solution and it is therefore assumed that free globin is stabilized in the cell in some way yet unknown.

Heywood and *Finch* (1970) studied the amount of free globin under conditions which influence haemoglobin synthesis. A low free-globin level was found in homozygous β-thalassaemia, in sickle-cell anaemia and iron-deficiency anaemia, while in anaemias not caused by impaired haemoglobin synthesis the amount of free globin was normal.

A surprising finding is the low free-globin level in iron-deficiency anaemia. In haem deficiency caused by iron deficiency we would rather expect an increase in free globin.

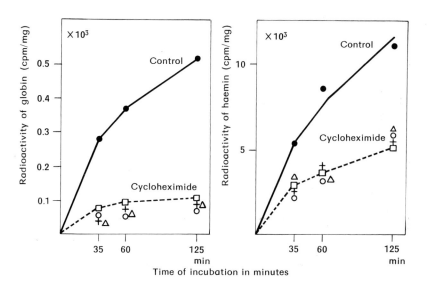

Fig. 46. Effect of cycloheximide on incorporation of glycine-2-^{14}C into globin and haem in rabbit reticulocytes. Concentrations of cycloheximide: △, 10^{-3}M; ○, 10^{-4}M; +, 10^{-5}M, □, 10^{-6}M; ●, control reticulocytes. (From *Neuwirt et al.*, 1969b. Reproduced with the permission of J. F. Lehmanns Verlag, Munich.)

There are several possible explanations for this. The increased amount of free proto-porphyrin which is a typical feature of these anaemias can combine with the accumulated globin and thus reduce the number of binding sites for haem. The haem deficiency may also activate cellular ribonuclease (*Burka*, 1968b) which may lead to earlier disintegration of ribosomes and to arrest of globin synthesis. Finally haem seem to be required during initiation of globin-chain synthesis (*see* p. 131).

The mechanism of regulation of haem synthesis by haem has been discussed in detail elsewhere (p. 82). This regulation comprises the inhibitory action of haem on iron uptake by the cell and the action of haem on the formation of ALA synthetase. It cannot be completely ruled out that haem also acts on other enzymes of porphyrin metabolism. Haem can also interfere with the transport of some substrates or enzymes across the mitochondrial membrane. The delayed haem synthesis in erythroid cells with inhibition of globin synthesis is explained by accumulation of free haem which in turn inhibits its own synthesis.

The experimental inhibition of haem or globin synthesis is a very convenient model for studying the mutual relations between haem and globin synthesis in intact cells. *Grayzel et al.* (1967) were the first to show that in reticulocytes incubated with

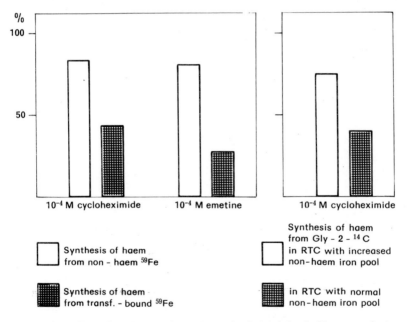

Fig. 47. The effect of inhibitors of protein synthesis (cycloheximide or emetine) on the utilization of transferin-bound ^{59}Fe and intracellular non-haem radioiron for haem synthesis; in the second part of the figure the effect of cycloheximide on glycine-2-^{14}C utilization for haem synthesis in reticulocytes with normal or elevated non-haem iron pool is compared. The results are expressed as percentages of control values. (From *Neuwirt et al.*, 1971.)

inhibitors of globin synthesis, cycloheximide or puromycin, haem synthesis is also greatly inhibited. These authors concluded that deficiency of globin for the association with haem leads to haem accumulation inside the cell. These findings were also confirmed in our laboratory (*Neuwirt et al.*, 1969b) (Fig. 46). Our results, however, did not confirm the hypothesis of *Grayzel* and co-workers that the synthesis of haem decreases due to ALA synthetase inhibition by the accumulated free haem. Our results suggest rather that haem inhibits the entry of iron into the cell by a feedback mechanism and thus reduces its own synthesis (*see* Fig. 31).

Some further experiments were performed to demonstrate that the reduced entry of iron into reticulocytes in the presence of free haem is a factor participating in the diminished haem synthesis during inhibited globin synthesis. The experiments revealed that in reticulocytes with an artificially raised content of non-haem iron the inhibition of haem synthesis by haem accumulating during inhibition of globin synthesis is much smaller than in normal reticulocytes. In normal reticulocytes incubated with cycloheximide haem synthesis is after one hour's incubation inhibited by as much as 60%, compared with control values, while in reticulocytes with an artificially raised non-haem iron pool haem synthesis assessed by incorporation of labelled glycine is inhibited by only 20 % or less (Fig. 47). These results indicate that the reduced supply of iron into reticulocytes with inhibited globin synthesis is of considerable importance for the reduction of haem synthesis.

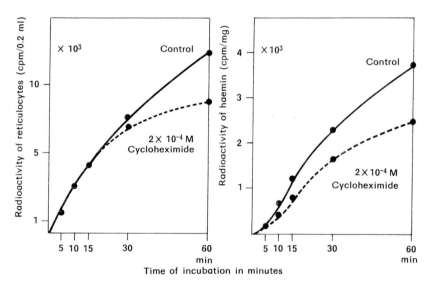

Fig. 48. Effect of cycloheximide on the reticulocyte radioiron uptake and on the incorporation of ^{59}Fe into haem. Radioiron and cycloheximide were added to the incubation mixture simultaneously. (From *Neuwirt et al.*, 1969b. Reproduced with the permission of J. F. Lehmanns Verlag, Munich.)

In subsequent experiments iron incorporation into reticulocytes with inhibited globin synthesis was studied in detail. The iron uptake by the cell does not differ from controls during the first 15 min but later begins to decline (Fig. 48). Similar results were obtained by *Fellicetti et al.* (1966). In our opinion these experiments can be interpreted in the sense that in reticulocytes uncommitted haem accumulates which later prevents further entry of iron into the cell. This mechanism, however, can hardly explain the very early inhibition of haem synthesis in reticulocytes which can already be detected 5 min after addition of cycloheximide.

HAEMOGLOBIN SYNTHESIS DURING MATURATION

During maturation cells pass through different number of mitoses. DNA synthesis ceases at the stage of polychromatophilic erythroblasts (*Borsook*, 1964; *Lajtha*, 1957). After cessation of DNA synthesis no further mitoses occur and the subsequent development involves the maturation of the orthochromatic erythroblasts into reticulocytes (*Grasso* and *Woodward*, 1967).

In mammals the nucleus disappears during maturation, while in birds and amphibians it remains even in circulating erythroblasts although no DNA, RNA or protein is synthesized there (*Grasso* and *Woodward*, 1966, *Harris H.*, 1967; *Scherrer*, 1967). Only in chick reticulocytes does RNA synthesis proceed, as can be shown by the action of actinomycin D (*Freedman et al.*, 1966).

The intensity of RNA synthesis is greatest in proerythroblasts and then declines continually (*Borsook*, 1964). At the stage of the orthochromatic erythroblast the intensity of RNA synthesis declines to 0.5% compared with the basophilic erythroblast (*Feinendegen et al.*, 1964). Rapidly labelled RNA molecules with a sedimentation constant from 4s to 150s were identified in the bone marrow of rats and ducks (*Gross* and *Goldwasser*, 1968, 1969; *Krantz* and *Goldwasser*, 1965; *Scherrer*, 1967). These rapidly labelled RNA molecules probably contain mRNA, rRNA and tRNA (*see also* p. 152).

After cessation of nucleic-acid synthesis, RNA which remains in erythroid cells controls the haemoglobin synthesis. mRNA is produced as long as the nucleus works. Otherwise the whole apparatus needed for protein synthesis is preserved. The intensity of protein synthesis as a whole during maturation declines only slightly, the main feature of maturation is, however, that haemoglobin synthesis replaces the synthesis of other proteins. Another factor contributing to haemoglobin accumulation is the breakdown of non-haemoglobin proteins (*Borsook*, 1964). Once formed haemoglobin remains in the cell until its lysis and finally accounts for more than 95% of the total protein in the cell (Fig. 49).

Haemoglobin can be estimated in sufficient amounts and with a sufficient sensitivity by means of microspectrophotometry and by cytochemical staining only at the stage of polychromatophilic erythroblasts (*Thorell*, 1947; *Ackerman*, 1962; *Grasso*

144

et al., 1963). Thorell's suggestion that intense haemoglobinization does not commence earlier than at the stage of the polychromatophilic erythroblast has now been fully confirmed. It must, however, be emphasized that even in earlier stages slow haemoglobin synthesis takes place and a very small amount of haemoglobin is already detectable in basophilic erythroblasts (*Thorell*, 1947; *Borsook et al.*, 1968a,b). Haemoglobin synthesis rapidly reaches its maximum at the stage of the polychromatophilic erythroblast and begins to decline in reticulocytes.

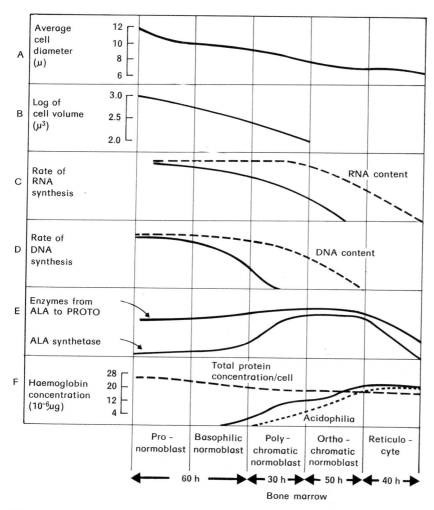

Fig. 49. Changes of various substances during erythroid differentiation and maturation. Substances listed in left-hand column are represented by corresponding solid black lines. Unless specified, graphs represent relative values. (From *Granick* and *Levere*, 1964. Reproduced with the permission of the authors and Grune and Stratton, Inc., New York.)

It is assumed that cessation of nucleic acid synthesis is due to the interaction of intranuclear haemoglobin and nucleohistone. This interaction leads then to condensation of the nuclear mass (*Stohlman et al.*, 1963, 1964; *Stohlman*, 1967, 1970b). The haemoglobin concentration is critical for this process and it seems that when its concentration in the cytoplasm is about 20%, nucleic-acid synthesis stops.

Yataganas et al. (1970) provided evidence for the hypothesis that the haemoglobin concentration plays an important role in the repression of DNA template activity for haemoglobin synthesis, in the same way as it does for DNA synthesis.

Assessment of the haemoglobin content in G_1-, S- and G_2- cells revealed that the amount of haemoglobin is greatest in the early stage S and is unaltered in the median phase S to phase G_2. It thus seems that haemoglobin is mainly synthesized during G_1 and probably during the initial stages of phase S.

The haemoglobin content does not increase in subsequent stages of phase S and G_2; on the other hand, throughout the interphase the dry matter content rises. This increase of dry matter content in phase S and G_2 is due to an enhanced synthesis of non-haem protein and nucleic-acid synthesis. In S- and G_2- cells the haemoglobin concentration declines gradually.

During the whole maturation process the haemoglobin content as well as its concentration increases. The enhanced haemoglobin synthesis takes place at the expense of the synthesis of other non-haem proteins. The dry matter of cells in G_1 gradually diminishes indicating that the cellular mass in erythroblasts does not completely double during the interphase. Every division thus involves a certain diminution of cellular mass in the G_1-phase. The haemoglobin content, however, increases progressively.

If the mean haemoglobin concentration rises above 22%, no more cells in phase S or G_2 are found. It is assumed that this increased concentration is the critical limit where no further DNA replication is possible and template activity of DNA for haemoglobin synthesis is completely repressed (*Yataganas et al.*, 1970).

The mechanism of this repression is not known. Haemoglobin can act indirectly by influencing the binding of DNA to protein. These reflections are based on findings of intranuclear haemoglobin and the fact that haemoglobin combines with DNA *in vitro*. *Harris* (1967) provided evidence that condensation of chromatin and arrest of RNA and DNA synthesis in the nuclei of bird erythrocytes need not necessarily be irreversible. After addition of nuclei from bird erythrocytes to HeLa cells the nucleus increased in size and RNA synthesis recommenced.

Glass et al. (1975a) investigated haem and globin synthesis in separated erythroid precursors of mice. They found that even in pronormoblasts there is a relatively high degree of incorporation of ^{59}Fe (Fig. 50) and glycine-^{14}C into haem and δ-amino-laevulinic acid synthetase is also well developed in the least mature cells. The greatest activity of haem synthesis was in basophilic and polychromatic normoblasts and declined with advancing maturation. On the other hand, haemoglobin synthesis

146

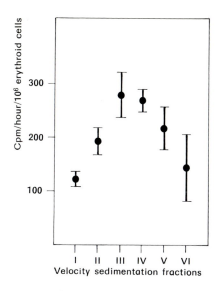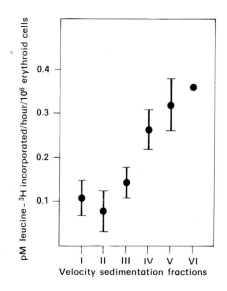

Fig. 50. ^{59}Fe incorporation into haem in the velocity sedimentation fractions. Results are means $\pm$ SE for six experiments. Fraction I contains the most immature cells, mainly pronormoblasts (67.5 %) and basophilic normoblasts (18 %), with only 14 % benzidine-positive cells. Fraction III contains primarily basophilic and polychromatic normoblasts, while fractions V and VI are composed largely of benzidine-positive cells. For details *see Glass et al.* (1975a). (Reproduced with the permission of the authors and the Rockefeller University Press, New York.)

Fig. 51. Leucine-^{3}H incorporation into haemoglobin in the velocity sedimentation fractions. Results are means $\pm$ SE for four experiments: those for fraction VI are from one experiment. The composition of the velocity sedimentation fractions is described in Fig. 50. For details *see Glass et al.* (1975a). (Reproduced with the permission of the authors and the Rockefeller University Press, New York.)

(measured by means of leucine-^{3}H) was very low in pronormoblasts and increased gradually (Fig. 51). It seems thus that haem synthesis in erythroid cells in the bone marrow appears at an earlier stage than haemoglobin synthesis. Although the rate of haem and haemoglobin syntheses differed, the synthesis of both these compounds could be considerably promoted by incubation with erythropoietin. The authors conclude that erythropoietin stimulates the biochemical differentiation in various stages of maturation.

DNA polymerase from rabbit reticulocytes has recently been isolated (*Byrnes et al.,* 1974). Its role in the cytoplasm of erythroid cells is, however, not quite clear. It is thought that this enzyme could be involved in cell differentiation.

Control of gene expression in mammalian cells is usually discussed in terms of transcription control in the nucleus and translation control in the cytoplasm. Translation control mechanisms are probably very important in higher organisms where it is assumed that there exists a considerable metabolic stability of mRNA in differen-

147

tiated mammalian cells. This assumption is based among other things on findings in reticulocytes which do not possess a nucleus and are thus unable to synthesize haemoglobin very actively. Administration of inhibitors of DNA-dependent RNA synthesis such as actinomycin D is often without effect on the synthesis of various enzymes; this is also used as evidence for the stability of mRNA. It cannot be ruled out, however, that mRNA is also continuously formed in the presence of actinomycin D, not from DNA but from RNA template. *Downey et al.* (1973) demonstrated in rabbit reticulocytes the presence of RNA polymerase which uses mRNA as a template for RNA synthesis. Evidence of RNA replicase in anucleated reticulocytes may represent an important mechanism during the flow of genetic information and another site of control for gene expression in the cytoplasm of higher organisms. Amplification of cytoplasmatic mRNA-dependent polymerase should render a considerable increase in specific protein synthesis possible without production of gene copies. The observation that RNA-dependent RNA polymerase is not inhibited by actinomycin D can explain the fact that actinomycin D does not influence haemoglobin synthesis in immature erythroid cells. It is of interest that this RNA polymerase is inhibited by haem in a concentration very close to that at which haem stimulates protein synthesis. In immature erythroid cells globin mRNA could serve not only as a template for globin synthesis but also as a template for RNA-dependent RNA polymerase. It cannot be ruled out that one of the regulatory roles of haem in maturing erythroid cells is to render possible preferential translation of mRNA for globin by haem inhibiting RNA polymerase.

6. DIFFERENTIATION OF ERYTHROID CELLS

Some cells of complex metazoan organisms are adapted to perform specialized functions. The progressive specialization in structure and function of cells is achieved by a process of differentiation. Since the genetic information in most cells of an organism is identical with that of every other cell, the tremendous diversity of cell phenotypes is due to the fact that each cell expresses only a limited amount of its full genetic potential. This means that different cell types express varying portions of their genome. Erythroid differentiation represents the expression of those parts of the cell genome that code for proteins (mainly haemoglobin) which define the cell as erythroid.

In higher chordates erythropoesis begins early in foetal life in the yolk sac and then shifts to the liver, spleen and bone marrow. Primitive yolk sac erythropoiesis is a transient process without the capacity of self-renewal or substained erythropoieses. The second or definitive erythroid cell line is mainly a product of hepatic erythropoiesis during the essential part of foetal life. This change in the type of erythroid cell line is accompanied by a change in the type of haemoglobin produced. In man primitive haemoglobin Gower is replaced by haemoglobin F when the site of erythropoiesis shifts to the liver.

The liver is also a transient haemopoietic site and is supplanted, even during foetal life, by the spleen and marrow which persist depending on the species as the sites of adult haematopoiesis. During human ontogeny haemoglobin F disappears and haemoglobins A and A_2 appear in increasing amounts. However, the switch from F to A production does not seem to be related to a change in the site of erythropoiesis (*Rifkind et al.*, 1974).

A comprehensive review of erythroid cell differentiation and haemoglobin synthesis during embryonic development has been published elsewhere (*Rifkind et al.*, 1974). In the following section an attempt will be made to discuss various aspects of erythroid differentiation in an adult organism. The main attention will be focused on the effect of erythropoietin and relevant data concerning the action of the hormone on foetal liver will also be presented.

ERYTHROID DIFFERENTIATION IN HAEMATOPOIETIC TISSUE AND THE INITIATION OF HAEMOGLOBIN SYNTHESIS

A simple calculation, based on the normal life span of red blood cells and their number in the human body, shows that in a normal person (70 kg), about 2×10^{11} erythrocytes have to be produced daily to maintain the steady state equilibrium of circulating erythrocytes. The mature erythrocytes are derived from a class of early undifferentiated cells, termed "stem cells", through a sequence of differentiation and proliferation. The erythroid cells share a common precursor cell with the myeloid and megakaryocytic series. This common precursor cell is called a pluripotent stem cell (*see Lajtha*, 1975). Intermediate between the pluripotent stem cell and recognizable erythroid cells is an unipotent stem cell which is committed to erythropoiesis (*see Lajtha*, 1975). Neither pluripotent stem cells nor cells committed to erythropoiesis have been morphologically characterized and these cells are defined according to their functions.

The mechanism by which the pluripotent stem cell is differentiated into precursor cells committed to erythropoiesis is still unknown. It has been suggested that the exposure to a specific haematopoietic inductive microenvironment results in differentiation of pluripotent stem cells into committed precursor cells (*Trentin*, 1970). There is also some evidence that androgen-derived steroids of 5-β-H configuration might be involved in the development of committed erythroid precursor cells from uncommitted stem cells (*Necheles*, 1971). The biochemical basis of differentiation of pluripotent stem cells into the committed compartment remains obscure.

The erythroid committed precursor cell responds to a humoral factor, erythropoietin, by differentiation into a "recognizable" erythroblast. There is evidence both *in vivo* and *in vitro* for the existence of a cell responsive to erythropoietin (ERC). In animals with suppressed erythropoietin production (e.g. hypertransfused mice) there is no morphological evidence of differentiated erythroid elements. The administration of erythropoietin to such animals stimulated the appearance of a new generation of early pronormoblasts (*Gurney et al.*, 1962). However, these newly differentiated erythroid cells do not originate directly from pluripotent stem cells (*Bruce* and *McCulloch*, 1964). Data assembled *in vitro* also indicate the existence of an erythroid committed precursor population (e.g. *Axelrad et al.*, 1974; *Mitchel* and *Adamson*, 1975; *Iscove*, 1975; *Iscove* and *Sieber*, 1975). It should be pointed out that erythropoietin is not only involved in the second-step differentiation of the erythropoietin-responsive cell into the erythron but it also seems to play a role in stimulating proliferation of ERC (*Reissman* and *Udupa*, 1972). Moreover, there are data suggesting that erythropoietin may affect already maturing erythroid elements (*see* p. 155).

Erythropoietin is absolutely essential for the normal production of red cells. It can be demonstrated in the urine of normal human beings and it may be obtained in large amounts from plasma or urine of anaemic animals or patients. The primary site of erythropoietin production is the kidney; erythropoietin production is controlled by the oxygen tension in the renal tissue (*Krantz* and *Jacobson*, 1970). Erythropoietin is a glycoprotein and the molecular weight of the native hormone is 46,000 daltons (*Goldwasser*, 1975a; 1975b).

MECHANISM OF ERYTHROPOIETIN ACTION

Erythropoietin induces second-step differentiation (*see* above) which means in biochemical terms the expression of genes that determine the synthesis of red-cell specific proteins, mainly haemoglobin. The mechanism of erythropoietin action has been studied using *in vitro* cultures of either adult rat and mouse bone marrow cells or foetal liver cells.

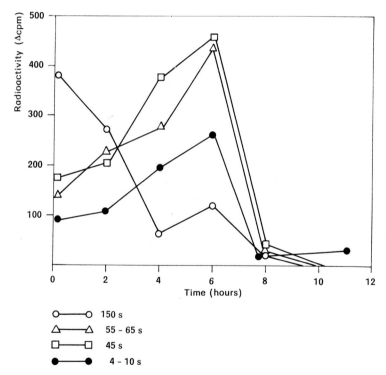

Fig. 52. Variations in rates of erythropoietin-stimulated RNA synthesis with time. Cultures containing $30 \cdot 10^6$ nucleated cells per ml in a total volume of 3.0 ml were preincubated for 7 hours, and then given 0.25 unit of erythropoietin/ml or an equal volume of medium. At each indicated time one control and one stimulated culture were pulsed for 15 min with uridine-^{3}H (2 µCi/ml) after which RNA was isolated. Details may be found in the original paper. (From *Gross* and *Goldwasser*, 1969. Reproduced with the permission of the American Chemical Society, Washington.)

151

The earliest detectable effect of erythropoietin on target cells is an increase in **RNA synthesis.** This effect of erythropoietin was demonstrated in rat bone marrow (*Krantz* and *Goldwasser*, 1965) as well as in foetal liver cells (*Paul* and *Hunter*, 1969; *Djaldetti et al.*, 1972) incubated *in vitro*. In both adult marrow cells (*Gross* and *Goldwasser*, 1969, 1971) and foetal tissues (*Nicol et al.*, 1972; *Maniatias et al.*, 1973; *Terada et al.*, 1975) erythropoietin stimulates a wide spectrum of RNA molecules sedimenting at 4s, 6s, 9s, 45s and 55 to 65s. Within several minutes of exposure of adult rat marrow cells *in vitro* to erythropoietin they synthesize a small amount of 150s RNA which is not present in control cells (*Gross* and *Goldwasser*, 1969). This RNA is confined to the nuclei of the marrow cells but its function is unknown. Very shortly after synthesis of 150s RNA is induced, heterogeneous nuclear RNA (55 to 65s) is formed as a result of erythropoietin action. This RNA seems to be a precursor to 9s globin mRNA (*see* p. 104). Thereafter the nuclear rRNA precursor (45s RNA) is produced and processed rRNA (18s and 28s RNA) and tRNA (4s) are formed. The sedimentation coefficient of 9s RNA suggests that this RNA may be the globin message (*Gross* and *Goldwasser*, 1969, 1971; *Goldwasser*, 1975b). This effect of erythropoietin on the synthesis of various types of RNA is shown in Fig. 52.

The first convincing evidence that erythropoietin stimulates globin mRNA synthesis came from studies conducted by *Terada et al.* (1972). These authors demonstrated that foetal mouse erythroid precursor cells, purified by immunolysis (*Cantor et al.*, 1972), do not contain any biologically active globin mRNA (i.e. translatable mRNA). Globin mRNA, translatable in a cell-free system (*see* p. 95), is first recognized between 5 and 10 hours after cultivation with erythropoietin, corresponding to the initiation of haemoglobin synthesis. Using the technique of hybridization with cDNA to globin mRNA, the same group of investigators ruled out the possibility that there could be a pool of non-translatable globin mRNA which accumulated during erythroid cell differentiation (*Ramirez et al.*, 1975). These hybridization techniques confirmed that globin mRNA is not present in the early precursor cells and appears after several hours of incubation with erythropoietin.

The above studies, however, did not make it possible to estimate the amount of globin mRNA in a given cell or to correlate changes in amounts of globin mRNAs with changes in the state of differentiation of the cell. Recently *Harrison et al.* (1973) described a method which allows detection of minute traces of globin mRNA in cytological specimens of cells. The method is based on *in situ* hybridization of globin messenger RNA to complementary DNA. It has been reported that only 2 per cent proerythroblasts from 11.5 day foetal mouse liver contain globin mRNA, demonstrated by using cDNA as a probe. As early as 1.5–2.5 h after commencement of treatment with erythropoietin *in vitro*, proerythroblasts accumulate globin mRNA (*Conkie et al.*, 1975). It may be suggested that in foetal mouse tissue erythropoietin initiates globin mRNA transcription in proerythroblasts. This conclusion can be extended to adult systems since after induction of a high level of erythropoietin *in vivo*, proerythroblasts in mouse spleen begin to accumulate globin mRNA (*Conkie et al.*, 1975). Data concerning the exact time of appearance of the first globin mRNA molecules in adult erythroid precursor cells after addition of erythropoietin *in vitro* are, however, still lacking. There are no data available concerning the appearance of globin mRNA in erythropoietin responsive cells. The transcription of the globin gene, as well as synthesis of other RNA species, is probably preceded by the activation of nuclear DNA-dependent RNA polymerase in erythroid precursor cells which were in contact with erythropoietin (*Piantadosi et al.*, 1976). Erythropoietin does not seem to induce *de novo* synthesis of RNA polymerases since inhibition of protein synthesis fails to prevent the hormone-mediated increase in RNA synthesis (*Gross* and *Goldwasser*, 1972).

Erythropoietin-mediated acceleration of RNA synthesis is not directly dependent on DNA synthesis. Inhibition of DNA synthesis with hydroxyurea, cytosine arabinoside, 5-fluorodeoxyuridine or hexachloriridate did not prevent an increase in RNA synthesis induced by erythropoietin in both normal adult marrow cells and foetal mouse liver (*Gross* and *Goldwasser*, 1970; *Djaldetti et al.*, 1972; *Nicol et al.*, 1972; *Datta* and *Dukes*, 1975). The situation is somewhat different in systems that do not contain differentiated erythroblasts. The early effect of erythropoietin on RNA transcription is also independent of DNA synthesis in erythropoietin responsive cells not contaminated with differentiated erythroid elements. 90-minute incubation of bone marrow containing only erythropoietin responsive cells with cytosine arabinoside, however, completely abolishes the erythropoietin effect on RNA synthesis. The possible interpretation of this finding proposed by *Bedard* and *Goldwasser* (1976) is as follows: cytosine arabinoside inhibits DNA synthesis and thus reduces the number of cells in the G_2-phase in which the precursors respond to erythropoietin.

Erythropoietin stimulates **DNA synthesis** in various haemopoietic culture systems (*Krantz* and *Jacobson*, 1970; *Dukes*, 1968a; *Paul* and *Hunter*, 1969; *Chui et al.*, 1971) but there are conflicting data concerning the onset of increased DNA synthesis. For example *Paul* and *Hunter* (1969) reported that 1 hour of exposure to erythropoietin stimulates DNA synthesis while *Chui et al.* (1971) observed that erythropoietin did not increase DNA synthesis before 10 hours of cultivation. Since erythropoietin-induced DNA synthesis is inhibited by inhibitors of either RNA or protein synthesis (*Gross* and *Goldwasser*, 1970), the increase in DNA synthesis appears to be relatively late event. Erythropoietin might directly increase the proliferation rate in the precursor compartment. However, the replication of erythropoietin-responsive cells may be stimulated indirectly as a result of decreased size of this compartment induced by erythropoietin.

Erythropoietin stimulates the **synthesis of cell membrane** components. This conclusion is based on the finding of increased incorporation of glucosamine into both stroma (*Dukes et al.*, 1964) and glycolipid (*Dukes*, 1968b). Erythropoietin-stimulated glucosamine incorporation into rat bone marrow cells apparently does not require increased DNA synthesis. It is tempting to speculate that increased incorporation of glucosamine represents *de novo* formation of receptors for the iron-transferrin complex on the membrane of precursor cells. There is some evidence that the transferrin membrane receptor is a glycoprotein (*Sly et al.*, 1975b). The building-up of these receptors may represent a prerequisite for the iron uptake needed by erythroid cells for the synthesis of haemoglobin. It should be noted that the effect of erythropoietin on cellular glucosamine uptake is apparent only after about 5 hours, while an increase in cellular iron uptake commences earlier (*see* below). However, the appearance of any biochemical response to erythropoietin depends on the sensitivity of the method applied. The sensitivity of methods used for estimation of various biochemical parameters may differ considerably.

Erythropoietin stimulates **iron incorporation** into bone-marrow cells (*Hrinda* and *Goldwasser*, 1969; *Storring* and *Fatih*, 1975). Erythropoietin-stimulated increase

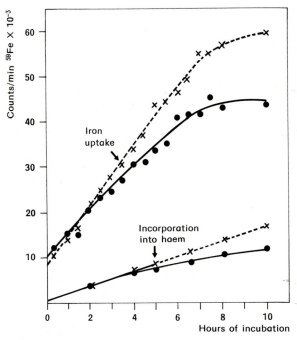

Fig. 53. Time course of ^{59}Fe uptake and incorporation into haem by marrow cells in Spinner flasks. Conditions of incubations: Medium, 47.5% newborn calf serum, 47.5% NCTC-109, 5% rat serum; vol., 30 ml per flask. Cell concentration was $1.4 \cdot 10^7$ nucleated cells per ml. ^{59}Fe was bound to rat serum (2 µCi per ml of medium). Erythropoietin concentration was 0.10 units/ml. Cells were added as 3 ml of concentrated suspension to 27 ml of medium at 37° containing all additions. ×——×, erythropoietin-stimulated cells; ●——●, control cells. (From *Hrinda* and *Goldwasser*, 1969. Reproduced with the permission of Elsevier/North-Holland Biomedical Press B. V., Amsterdam.)

154

in cellular iron uptake, commencing notably early, precedes stimulated haem synthesis (Fig. 53). This leads to iron accumulation in ferritin, which is apparent within 1 hour, and later in a low molecular weight fraction. This erythropoietin-enhanced iron uptake into ferritin, however, seems to be due to increased transport of iron into the cell rather than to a direct effect on ferritin synthesis (*Storring* and *Fatih*, 1975). It is not known whether increased iron uptake after erythropoietin is due to the stimulation of iron-transferrin uptake or results from the increased release of iron from transferrin. There is some indirect evidence supporting the latter possibility since the effect of erythropoietin on iron incorporation into ferritin and low molecular weight iron fraction can be mimicked by isonicotinic acid hydrazide (INH) (*Storring* and *Fatih*, 1975). INH is known to decrease the intracellular haem pool and thus stimulates the rate of iron release from transferrin (*see* p. 45). It should be pointed out that such an early effect of erythropoietin on the iron metabolism in bone-marrow cells probably represents the effect of hormone on erythroblasts that are already differentiated. Erythropoietin added to cultures from hypertransfused rats (which do not contain differentiated erythroid elements) increased the rate of iron uptake after a lag of 7 hours and the rate of haemoglobin synthesis was stimulated after a lag of 12 hours (*Gross* and *Goldwasser*, 1971).

The increased intracellular iron level is of considerable importance for further differentiation and maturation processes. Iron is not only a substrate for haem synthesis but also seems to increase the activity of ALA synthetase by accelerating the formation of this enzyme, probably at the translation level (*Takaku* and *Nakao*, 1971). Moreover, the iron requirement for DNA synthesis, mitosis and cell division in bone marrow has been described (*Hershko et al.*, 1970; *Van der Weyden et al.*, 1972).

Following this early increase in iron uptake, an increase in iron incorporation into haem occurs. This effect of erythropoietin is due to hormone-stimulated synthesis of enzymes involved in **haem synthesis** (*Nakao et al.*, 1968; *Bottomley* and *Smithee*, 1969). Erythropoietin administered *in vivo* to polycythaemic mice stimulates consecutively the activity of ALA synthetase, ALA dehydrase and haem synthetase (*Nakao et al.*, 1968).

In summary, erythropoietin affects commited erythroid precursor cells and induces in these cells the expression of those genes, the products of which (such as haemoglobin) define the cell as erythroid. However, the exact sequence of events which procede the synthesis of the complete haemoglobin molecule has still not been completely elucidated. In marrow cells from polycythaemic mice (which contain erythropoietin-responsive cells but not differentiated erythroid elements), one of the first effects of erythropoietin is the initiation of 9s RNA synthesis which occurs as early as 1 hour after erythropoietin. In the same system erythropoietin stimulates haemoglobin synthesis after a lag of 12 hours. *Gross* and *Goldwasser* (1971) therefore suggested that some control mechanism operates between the transcription of 9 s RNA, the presumed globin messenger, and its translation. This concept was, however, criticized since 9s RNA appearing after erythropoietin need not necessarily represent the globin messenger. Moreover, recent studies with the differentiation of foetal erythroid cells provide no evidence of a pool of non-translatable globin mRNA (*Ramirez et al.*, 1975). In any case one of the first effects of erythropoietin is the stimulation of globin mRNA synthesis, although this event is preceded by increased production of various types of RNAs which might include HnRNA containing globin mRNA. It is not clear whether other cell functions (e.g. increased activity of the machinery for haem synthesis) depend directly on erythropoietin or are activated secondarily. For example one can envisage that erythropoietin triggers the globin mRNA appearance and the first globin chains combine with pre-existing haem (note: a low level of haem synthesis must already occur in stem cells). The decreased level of intracellular haem might induce the synthesis of ALA synthetase (*see* p. 73) and facilitate the release of iron from transferrin (*see* p. 45).

Another question is the way in which the erythroid precursor cell recognizes erythropoietin and what are the molecular mechanisms transporting the signal to the cell nuclei. *Chang et al.* (1974) presented data suggesting that there is a protein on the external surface of the erythropoietin responsive cell which is required for the erythropoietin effect on RNA synthesis. This erythropoietin receptor can be destroyed by trypsin treatment but it may be resynthesized by the cells if protein synthesis is allowed to proceed.

Erythropoietin does not pass through the cell membrane nor do isolated nuclei respond to added erythropoietin (*Goldwasser*, 1975b; *Chang* and *Goldwasser*, 1973), so there should be a secondary signal operating between cell surface recognition of extracellular erythropoietin and the cell nucleus. *Chang* and *Goldwasser* (1973) have demonstrated a **cytoplasmic fraction** from rat marrow cells exposed to erythropoietin which stimulated RNA synthesis by marrow-cell nuclei. This factor seems to be protein but it is generated in the absence of protein synthesis. The formation of this active cytoplasmic fraction is specific for bone-marrow cells; however, the marrow-cell cytoplasmic factor also stimulates RNA synthesis by liver and kidney nuclei.

The requirement of such an intermediate of erythropoietin action on cell nuclei led to speculations that cyclic nucleotides might be responsible for transferring the signal. However, erythropoietin does not affect the level of cyclic AMP in foetal rat-liver erythroid cells after 5 or 30 minutes where a major effect on haemoglobin synthesis is later observed (*Graber et al.*, 1973, 1974). Similarly, neither cyclic AMP nor cyclic GMP stimulate haemoglobin synthesis in rat marrow cells (*Graber et al.*, 1972; *Goldwasser*, 1975b). A more recent report indicates that the lack of cyclic AMP effect on haemoglobin synthesis may be related to the mammalian species studies. Cyclic AMP does not stimulate haem synthesis in rat, mouse, nor guinea-pig bone-marrow cells. On the other hand, cyclic AMP stimulates haem synthesis in cultures of human, sheep, rabbit and canine cells (*Brown* and *Adamson*, 1974). The hypothesis that cyclic nucleotides might mediate the action of erythropoietin at the cellular level should be therefore reconsidered.

The whole process of **erythroid cell differentiation** may be, according to *Goldwasser* (Fig. 54), divided into three distinct phases: sensitization, induction and specialization.

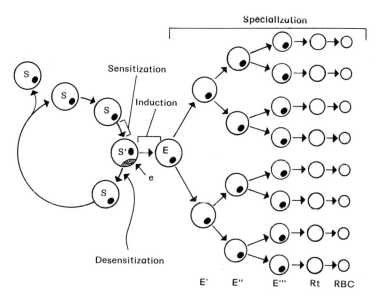

Fig. 54. Proposed division of erythropoietin action into phases. S represents erythropoietin sensitive stem cell; S', sensitized cell; E, induced cell; E', E", E''' later stages of erythroid differentiation. Rt. reticulocyted; RBC, red cell. The stippled areas represent an attachment site for erythropoietin. e. (From *Goldwasser*, 1975b. Reproduced with the permission of the Federation of American Societies for Experimental Biology, Bethesda.)

Sensitization is the process by which cells synthesize receptors for erythropoïetin. Induction represents the primary action of erythropoietin on the cell nucleus. As already discussed in detail, erythropoietin induces indirectly those transcriptional processes (i.e. RNA synthesis) required for haemoglobin synthesis. In the phase of specialization all the biochemical and morphological events following induction take place. These events include various functions such as iron transport and glucosamine incorporation, synthesis of enzymes of the haem synthetic pathway, globin synthesis, the formation of the complete haemoglobin molecule, and the formation of specific membrane antigens. On the other hand, during the process of specialization some of the functions — characteristic for the precursor cell stage — disappear.

ERYTHROID DIFFERENTIATION WITHOUT ERYTHROPOIETIN

In 1957 *Friend* described a virus that induced leukaemia in mice. Part of this disease was intensive erythropoiesis which resembled erythraemic myelosis in man. *Mirand* (1965, 1967) isolated a polycytheamia-inducing virus from some passage lines of Friend virus. Contrary to normal erythropoiesis, which is maintained by erythropoietin, virus-induced erythropoiesis is apparently independent of this humoral factor (*Mirand et al.*, 1971).

In tissue cultures of cells isolated from virus-induced leukaemia there is apparent differentiation to erythroid line (*Friend et al.*, 1966) and Friend-virus-induced leukaemic cells synthesize small amounts of haemoglobin in tissue cultures (*Scher et al.*, 1971). In the presence of dimethylsulfoxide (DMSO) these cells are stimulated to differentiate along the erythroid pathway and to form large amounts of haemo-

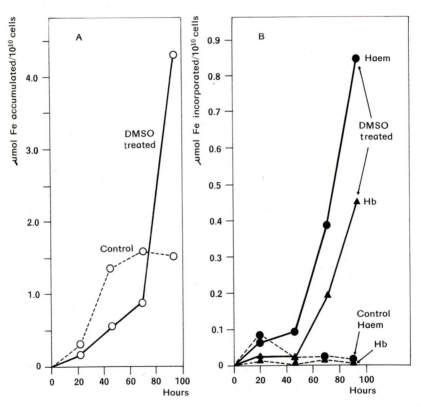

Fig. 55. Effect of dimethyl sulfoxide (DMSO) on the rate of cellular iron accumulation (A) and the rates of incorporation of iron into haem and haemoglobin (B). Details of experiments and methods used may be found in the original paper. (From *Friend et al.*, 1971. Reproduced with the permission of the authors and the National Academy of Sciences, Washington.)

globin (Fig. 55) (*Friend et al.*, 1971). This system is therefore useful for analyzing the mechanisms of control and differentiation of haemoglobin formation.

Ebert and *Ikawa* (1974) have reported that an early rise in ALA synthetase (by the 2nd day) occurred in DMSO-treated cells. Thereafter DMSO induces ALA dehydrase, uroporphyrinogen synthetase and consequently haem synthetase which seems to rise 4 days after treatment (*Sassa et al.*, 1975). These data suggest that a sequential gene activation of enzymes in the biosynthetic haem pathway may occur to bring about erythroid cell differentiation (Fig. 56).

Various Friend cell lines have also been used for studying the mechanisms of control of globin mRNA formation after DMSO treatment. The results suggest that different

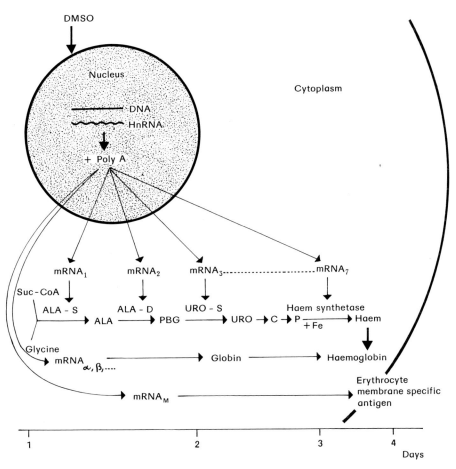

Fig. 56. A schematic representation of erythroid differentiation in Friend leukaemia cells. Time scale indicates approximate number of days after DMSO addition. (From *Sassa et al.*, 1975. Reproduced with the permission of the authors and University of Tokyo Press, Tokyo.)

159

control mechanisms are operating in various Friend cell lines. For example an un-induced clone of the Friend erythroleukaemic cells (T-3 C 12) contained virtually no globin mRNA. Globin mRNA increased markedly after DMSO treatment (*Ross et al.*, 1972b). Untreated M2 cells contain globin mRNA sequences in nuclear RNA and also in cytoplasmic RNA but in cytoplasmic RNA the globin mRNA concentration is much lower. After treating clone M2 cells with DMSO for 5 days, the globin mRNA content of nuclear RNA increased abour 6-times whereas the globin mRNA content of polyribosomes increased 50 to 100 times (*Gilmour et al.*, 1974). Thus in M2 cells DMSO seems to increase the rate of transcription from chromatin rather than to initiate it. Moreover, in this cell type there is also control at a post-transcriptional level which explains the discrepancies between the nuclear and cytoplasmic changes in the globin mRNA concentration. On the other hand, in clone 707 of the Friend cell control of haemoglobin synthesis is mediated almost entirely by post-transcriptional events (*Harrison et al.*, 1974). These results suggest that Friend leukaemia cells represent an excellent model for studying concerted mechanisms during early erythroid maturation but probably cannot be used for the study of the initial step of erythropoiesis.

7. ANAEMIAS DUE TO DISORDERS OF HAEMOGLOBINIZATION

A reduction of the haemoglobin level induces an increase in bone marrow cell proliferation and red cell production. The response of erythroid elements in bone marrow to erythropoietic stimulation depends on various factors such as the severity of anaemia, the production of erythropoietin, the integrity of the haemopoietic inductive microenvironment, the availability of essential substrates and the specific characteristics of the anaemia (*Hillman*, 1970).

One of the most important factors which determine the response of bone marrow to anaemia is the iron supply to bone marrow (Table 15). Proliferation of red cell precursors in bone marrow can reach its maximum capacity only when there is an adaquate iron supply. Patients with iron deficiency respond to a considerable re-

Table 15

Marrow production response*

Disorder	Iron supply	Marrow expansion	Serum iron (µg%)	Maximum production (X's normal)
Iron deficiency	Food iron	0	10 – 40	1.0 – 1.5
Normal	RE cell iron stores	0	30 – 70	2.0 – 3.5
Haemochromatosis	RE cell plus parenchymal iron stores	0	70 – 200	4.5 – 5.0
Haemolytic anaemia	Increased red cell destruction or senescent red cell infusions	+ or + +	100 – 250	3.5 – 6.0
Normal		0	200 – 300	6.0 – 7.5
Thalassaemia	Ineffective erythropoiesis	+ + +	100 – 300	6.0 – 10.0
Pernicious anaemia	plus adult cell haemolysis	0	100 – 300	2.5 – 7.5

*Haematocrit 20–30%.
(From *Hillman*, 1969. Reproduced with the permission of the author and the New York Academy of Sciences, New York.)

161

duction of the haematocrit only by an inadequate increase in red cell production. The reason for inadequate proliferation of bone marrow cells in iron deficiency is probably reduced DNA synthesis due to bone marrow iron deficiency. It has long been known that patients with haemolytic anaemia with a maximum iron supply from haemolysed red cells can increase the production in bone marrow 5 to 7 times. A maximum proliferation of bone marrow was described in patients with thalassaemia (Table 15).

In anaemia maturation processes in bone marrow are also altered. After maximum erythroid stimulation in experimental animals reticulocytes are produced which are twice the size of normal red cells (*Brecher* and *Stohlman*, 1961, 1962). Mature cells which develop from these reticulocytes are macrocytes and have a reduced life span. This macrocytic response may also be induced by the administration of exogenous erythropoietin (*Stohlman et al.*, 1963). The assumption was expressed that this macrocytic response to severe anaemia develops as a result of the formation of endogenous erythropoietin and is proportional to the intensity of the erythropoietic stimulus. These large reticulocytes have a much more active haemoglobin synthesis (*Borssok et al.*, 1962) and have a large amount of RNA in the cytoplasm and therefore it is assumed that they are directly derived from nucleated basophilic erythroblasts or very young polychromatic erythroblasts (*Borsook et al.*, 1962; *Seno*, 1966).

An exception in this relationship of cell size to the severity of anaemia is iron-deficiency anaemia. In severe iron deficiency microcytes are produced even after administration of large doses of exogenous erythropoietin (*Stohlman et al.*, 1963). Cell size thus does not depend only on the amount of endogenous or exogenous erythropoietin but also on the availability of iron for haemoglobin synthesis.

From this it follows that erythropoietin initiates haemoglobin synthesis and the prerequisite of its maximum rate is an adequate supply of substrates. If the haemoglobin concentration reaches a critical level, nucleic acid synthesis is inhibited by a feedback mechanism and thus further division is arrested (*Stohlman et al.*, 1963). A more detailed description of the mechanism of action of high haemoglobin concentrations on nucleic acid synthesis has already been presented (*see* p. 146). Rapid haemoglobinization thus determines the number of cell divisions in the erythroid compartment. Erythropoietin accelerates haemoglobinization and reduces the time interval needed to attain the critical cytoplasmatic haemoglobin concentration. As a result of this the terminal division is eliminated and macrocytosis develops.

When haemoglobin synthesis is reduced, as e.g. in iron deficiency, the period before the critical cytoplasmatic haemoglobin concentration is reached, is prolonged. Therefore further mitoses occur and microcytosis develops (*Moores et al.*, 1963; *Stohlman et al.*, 1973).

The haemoglobin molecule is made up of two components: haem, the synthesis of which is completed in mitochondria, and four globin chains which are synthesized in ribosomes. The formation of the two components is closely coordinated by two main control mechanisms. The initiation of globin synthesis on ribosomes is dependent on haem availability and, on the other hand, haem inhibits its own synthesis by a feedback mechanism (*see* p. 135). This means practically that the primary disorder in the synthesis of either haem or globin is always associated with a decline in the formation of the whole haemoglobin molecule.

Reduced haemoglobin formation may thus be due to impaired haem or impaired globin formation. One of the reasons for reduced haem synthesis is a limited substrate supply for the formation of the prosthetic haemoglobin group. Haem is formed by an intricate synthesis from glycine, succinyl coenzyme A and iron. It has not been observed that haem formation declines as a result of a reduced supply or formation of the former two substances. On the other hand, iron deficiency is the most frequent cause of reduced haemoglobinization of erythroid cells. The second basic cause of reduced haem synthesis is the deficiency of some enzyme needed for protoporphyrin and haem formation.

Reduced haemoglobinization of erythroid cells may also occur when the synthesis of globin chains is unbalanced. An unbalanced synthesis of globin chains is found in thalassaemia which is a heterogeneous group of genetically conditioned disorders of impaired synthesis of globin chains. In certain forms of thalassaemia the synthesis of some types of chains is completely lacking, in other forms these chains are synthesized at a considerably reduced rate.

In subsequent paragraphs the aetiopathogenesis of anaemias caused by reduced rate of haemoglobin formation will be discussed. The result of the reduced rate of haemoglobin formation in the developing erythroid cell is a reduced haemoglobin concentration in the mature erythrocyte. These anaemias are therefore called hypochromic.

HYPOCHROMIC ANAEMIAS DUE TO IMPAIRED HAEM SYNTHESIS

HYPOCHROMIC ANAEMIAS CAUSED BY A REDUCED IRON SUPPLY INTO ERYTHROID TISSUE

Iron-deficiency anaemia

Iron-deficiency anaemia is one of the most common diseases and it is estimated that it affects hundreds of milions of people. It results from a disbalance between iron intake and losses. There are three stages of iron deficiency. The first stage is iron depletion or sideropenia, the second stage is described as iron-deficient erythropoiesis and the third stage is iron-deficiency anaemia (*Finch*, 1970; *Jacobs*, 1974). It must be realized that marked peripheral blood changes are found only in the third stage.

The first stage, iron depletion, is characterized by a reduced amount of iron in depots, the absence of haemosiderin in bone marrow reticuloendothelial cells and enhanced iron absorption (unless the impaired absorption is the inducing cause of iron deficiency). If iron depletion persists, after the iron reserves have been exhausted, the plasma iron level declines, the transferrin saturation drops below 18% (*Bothwell* and *Finch*, 1962). At the same time the number of sideroblasts declines (50% of normal erythroblasts contain iron granules and are therefore called sideroblasts). The decline of sideroblasts below the critical level of 10% is an indication of reduced iron supply into the erythroid cells of the bone marrow (*Bainton* and *Finch*, 1964) (Table 16).

Table 16
Laboratory measurements in iron deficiency

Measurement	Response time	Use	Limitations
Transferrin Fe sat. <16%	Hours	Best screening test for iron deficiency anaemia	Does not detect changes in iron stores and is not specific for iron deficiency (down in inflammation)
Sideroblast count <10%	Hours	Best measure of adequacy of cellular iron supply for haemoglobin synthesis	Affected by abnormalities in haemoglobin synthesis as well as in iron supply. It is difficult to perform and evaluate quantitatively
Protoporphyrin >50 μg/100 ml rbc	Days to weeks	Demonstrates inadequate iron supply to normoblasts	Not specific for iron deficiency anaemia (increased in inflammation)
Iron absorption increased	Days	The most quantitative method of evaluating iron balance in large group studies	An indirect measurement not specific for iron stores and not applicable to ill subjects
Marrow haemosiderin decreased or absent	Weeks or months	Most useful method for evaluating the iron status of the anaemic patient, especially in differentiating iron deficiency from inflammation	Not conveniently performed on well subjects and not quantitative
MCHC <30%	Months	Demonstrates decreased haemoglobin synthesis by the individual cell	Not present in early iron deficiency anaemia and not specific for iron deficiency (found in other blocks in haemoglobin synthesis)

(From *Finch*, 1970. Reproduced with the permission of the author and CIBA-GEIGY Ltd., Basle.)

164

During the gradual development of iron deficiency in the organism no changes in the peripheral red cells are found at first. Initially a condition develops where erythropoiesis is limited by iron and in that case the proliferation in bone marrow is also limited, while there is no haemoglobin deficiency in individual cells. Only later is the haemoglobin formation in the erythroid cell reduced resulting in iron deficiency anaemia. Initially, the anaemia is normocytic and normochromic and only later develops into microcytic hypochromic anaemia. According to *Finch* (1969) more than half the patients in whom erythropoiesis is limited by iron have no apparent iron deficiency changes in their peripheral red cells. If iron deficiency develops very rapidly as a result of a major blood loss, the anaemia is at first macrocytic (*see* response of erythropoiesis to anaemia, p. 162).

In iron deficiency anaemia in erythroblasts the rate of haem and globin formation declines. The disorder of haem formation is primary but not only because the essential substrate — iron — is lacking. Iron is also essential for optimum porphyrin synthesis and therefore when it is deficient, porphyrin synthesis is reduced (*Lichtmann* and *Feldmann*, 1967; *Prato et al.*, 1968). It must, however, be emphasized that in iron deficiency anaemias free protoporphyrin in red cells rises as a result of the disbalance between porphyrin synthesis and iron supply (*Dagg et al.*, 1966). Iron supply into erythroid cells is reduced more than the rate of protoporphyrin synthesis. Because protoporphyrin is lost from circulating red cells only very slowly, its level in red cells is a very accurate indicator of the degree of iron deficiency (Table 16).

It seems that iron deficiency alone limits proliferation. *Hershko et al.* (1970) demonstrated a considerable decline in the nucleic acid content of bone marrow cells and at the same time inhibition of thymidine-^{3}H incorporation into DNA in the bone marrow of patients with chronic iron deficiency (Table 17). This finding explains

Table 17

Thymidine-^{3}H and uridine-5-^{3}H incorporation into nucleic acids*

	Thymidine-^{3}H into DNA				Uridine-5-^{3}H into RNA			
	cpm after 60 min incubation		cpm/hour		cpm after 60 min incubation		cpm/hour	
	Mean	±S.D.	Mean	±S.D.	Mean	±S.D.	Mean	±S.D.
Normal control	1,400	245	600	176	500	48	800	124
Iron-deficient	500	73	120	21	510	67	700	106
After iron therapy	1,200	185	400	83	720	163	640	127

* cpm 10^9 nucleated cells.
(From *Hershko et al.*, 1970. Reproduced with the permission of authors and the Grune and Stratton, Inc., New York.)

why production of erythroid cells in patients with iron deficiency anaemia can increase one and a half times compared with normal subjects, while in haemolytic anaemia the production can be increased as much as seven fold.

The findings of *Hershko et al.* (1970) contribute to the suggestion that in iron-deficiency anaemia defective erythroid cells are formed. *Hershko* and co-workers observed an increased intracellular breakdown of RNA in bone marrow cells during chronic iron deficiency. It has been known for some time that iron deficiency is associated with the disaggregation of polyribosomes in reticulocytes (p. 129). When reticulocyte polyribosomes are disaggregated, some kinds of RNA are probably more susceptible to the effect of ribonuclease. Disorders of the nucleic acid metabolism also cause a considerable reduction of protein synthesis in bone-marrow cells. The synthesis of several important enzymes is inhibited, amongst others important enzymes of the biosynthetic porphyrin chain (*Lichtmann* and *Feldmann*, 1967; *Takaku* and *Nakao*, 1971).

In hypochromic microcytic anaemia which develops during prolonged iron deficiency the volume of the red cells as well as the amount of haemoglobin within the red cell and the haemoglobin concentration in the red cells diminish. The reduced haemoglobin concentration in red cells is the cause of the impaired structural integrity of the cells and thus the viability of the red blood cells declines. However, it cannot be ruled out that the reduced life span of hypochromic erythrocytes is connected with the other biochemical disorders mentioned above. Ineffective erythropoieses, which accompanies hypochromic iron-deficiency anaemia, can be explained in a similar way.

If we thus summarize the pathogenesis of iron-deficiency anaemia, we can see that iron deficiency prevents optimum haemoglobin synthesis in erythroblasts and reduces the ability of bone marrow to respond to anaemia by an increased production of erythroid cells. In addition there is an increased destruction of immature erythroblasts in bone marrow (ineffective erythropoiesis) and also partly a somewhat shorter life span as a result of haemoglobin deficiency and other biochemical disorders.

Among laboratory findings the lower plasma iron levels, the decline in the percentage of transferrin saturation with iron and the absolute rise of the transferrin level are important. Recently the reduction of the plasma ferritin level has also been considered an important indicator of iron deficiency (*Addison et al.*, 1972; *Jacobs et al.*, 1972; *Jacobs*, 1974). In the red cells the haemoglobin concentration (MCHC) declines below 30% and the free protoporphyrin level rises. Ferrokinetic investigations reveal a more rapid clearance rate of iron from plasma and a greater proportion of plasma iron is utilized for erythropoiesis.

Congenital atransferrinaemia

In this rare disease the specific binding protein for iron, transferrin, which is indispensible for the physiological iron supply into erythroid cells, is lacking. This rare congenital disorder was described by *Heilmayer et al.* (1961), *Čáp et al.* (1968) and *Goya et al.* (1972). In bone marrow sideroblasts are completely lacking and liver biopsy reveals severe siderosis. Hypochromic anaemia develops after birth and is completely refractory to any iron therapy. The administration of transferrin, however, leads to a considerable increase in the haemoglobin level.

The detection of complete atransferrinaemia also helped to answer some theoretical problems of iron metabolism. It was revealed that transferrin is not essential for iron absorption. On the other hand, this disease confirmed that iron can be supplied to erythroid cells only via transferrin (*see also* p. 16).

Hypochromic anaemia as a result of reduced iron release from reticuloendothelial cells

In infections, malignant conditions, severe allergic inflammations or rheumatic disease there is a considerable discrepancy between iron accumulation in reticulo-endothelial cells and the low iron content of erythroblasts. In infectious conditions it was shown that there is an impaired iron release from reticuloendothelial cells to transferrin (*Haurani et al.*, 1965) and this leads to a reduced iron concentration in plasma and to the development of hypochromic anaemia. However, in infections the pathogenesis of anaemia is more complex since there is evidence of increased red cell destruction.

Copper deficiency

In experimental animals copper deficiency produces hypochromic microcytic anaemia (*Lahey et al.*, 1952; *Cartwright et al.*, 1956). So far in man anaemia caused by copper deficiency has not been described. *Goodman* and *Dallman* (1969) provided evidence that copper plays a part in the intracellular iron transport into mitochondria where iron combines with protoporphyrin. In some animals with copper deficiency inhibition of cytochrome oxidase − an important enzyme in oxidative phospohorylations − has also been described (*Dallman* and *Loskutoff*, 1967). It is well known that iron release from transferrin and its entry into mitochondria depends on intact electron transport (*see* p. 22).

SIDEROBLASTIC ANAEMIAS

Sideroblastic anaemia is the term used to describe a heterogeneous group of anaemias of different aetiology having some features in common. These common characteristics of sideroblastic anaemias comprise hypochromic erythrocytes, a raised serum iron level, a raised saturation of transferrin and finally the presence of patholo-gical or so-called ringed sideroblasts in bone marrow. A characteristic feature is also erythroid hyperplasia of bone marrow (*Mollin* and *MacGibbon*, 1972; *Sullivan* and *Weintraub*, 1973; *Cartwright* and *Deiss*, 1975). In the cytoplasm of sideroblasts there are numerous iron-containing granules frequently surrounding the nuclei

167

in a ring. These are mitochondria filled with non-haem iron. In this respect these pathological sideroblasts differ from sideroblasts which are present in normal bone marrow where 20–80% of the nucleated red cells have iron-containing granules. Iron in these normal sideroblasts is in the form of ferritin and can be stained with Prussian blue; under normal conditions the bone marrow cells do not contain more than four granules. The number of these sideroblasts is directly proportional to the percentage of transferrin saturation with iron (*Bainton* and *Finch*, 1964).

In patients with sideroblastic anaemia iron accumulates in mitochondrial cristae and so far it has not been possible to prove that the iron is in the form of ferritin. Mitochondria damaged by iron are swollen. In the bone marrow of patients with refractory sideroblastic anaemia about 40–70% of the normoblasts are ringed sideroblasts. In some other types of sideroblastic anaemias this percentage is lower.

Sideroblastic anaemias are thus characterized by excessive iron accumulation in mitochondria. This iron is not used for haem synthesis.

In the pathogenesis of the majority of sideroblastic anaemias the most important part is played by the reduced rate of haem synthesis. Most frequently the activity of δ-aminolaevulinic acid synthetase is reduced. This is the key enzyme of porphyrin synthesis and determines the rate of protoporphyrin production (*Aoki et al.*, 1974). Defects of uroporphyrinogen decarboxylase (*Kushner* and *Barbuto*, 1974) and of haem synthetase (*Vogler* and *Mingiolli*, 1968) have also been described.

In erythroid cells of patients with sideroblastic anaemia the rate of globin formation also declines (*White et al.*, 1971). This decline is, however, secondary and results from the primary inhibition of haem synthesis (*see* p. 129).

The deficiency of a certain enzyme of porphyrin synthesis may be genetic or may be produced by some substances which interfere in particular with the metabolism of vitamin B_6 which, in the form of pyridoxal phosphate, is essential for the normal activity of δ-aminolaevulinic acid synthetase. Sideroblastic anaemia was experimentally induced in animals and observed in man after administration of isoniazide (INH) (*Hines* and *Grasso*, 1970; *Harlys et al.*, 1965), alcohol (*Grasso* and *Hines*, 1969; *Eichner* and *Hillman*, 1971), cycloserine (*Hines* and *Grasso*, 1970), pyrazinamide and lead (*Jensen* and *Moreno*, 1964). The majority of these substances inhibit the activity of ALA synthetase, while lead inhibits the biosynthesis of haem at several sites. Alcohol inhibits the biosynthesis of pyridoxal-5-phosphate from pyridoxine by inhibiting pyridoxal kinase (*Hines*, 1969) or promotes the degradation of pyridoxal-5-phosphate by activation of pyridoxal-phosphate phosphatase (*Lumeng* and *Li*, 1974). Isoniazide, cycloserine and pyrazinamide inhibit reactions catalyzed by pyridoxal phosphate (*Holtz* and *Palm*, 1974). It was demonstrated that INH inhibits pyridoxal kinase *in vivo* (*Haut et al.*, 1975). It seems that to inhibit pyridoxal kinase some INH metabolite must accumulate in the cell. Chloramphenicol inhibits mitochondrial protein synthesis in general and after its administration the activity of ALA synthetase (*Rosenberg* and *Marcus*, 1974) and haem synthetase (*Manyan*

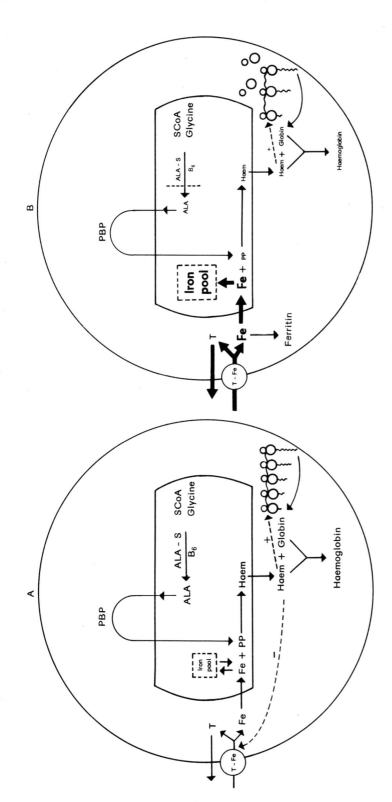

Fig. 57. Modification of the *Cartwright* and *Deiss* (1975) scheme of Intramitochondrial Iron Pathways. A – The availability of iron for mitochondria (oval area inside cell) depends on the rate of dissociation of iron from transferrin. This process, which might take place either on the cell membrane or in the cell interior (*see* p. 17), is limited by the level of uncommitted haem. B – Disturbance of intracellular iron metabolism as well as the defect in globin synthesis (*see* p. 129) caused by a decrease in uncommitted haem pool (due to an enzymatic block). Note: there is also slight iron incorporation into ferritin under normal conditions (not shown in the figure). Fe represents iron, T transferrin, PP protoporphyrin, SCoA succinyl CoA, ALA-S δ-aminolevulinic acid synthetase, B₆ pyridoxal-5′-phosphate and PBP the porphyrin biosynthetic pathway.

169

et al., 1972) declines. The majority of these sideroblastic anaemias responds favourably to pyridoxine administration although very rarely they are caused by dietary vitamin B$_6$ deficiency.

Kark et al. (1975) found that patients with so-called idiopathic refractory sideroblastic anaemia have an impaired vitamin B$_6$ metabolism in their erythrocytes. In these sideroblastic anaemias the synthesis of pyridoxal phosphate from pyridoxal and pyridoxine is enhanced, in contrast to the types of sideroblastic anaemia of toxic origin mentioned above which are associated e.g. with alcoholism or administration of IHN, where the synthesis of pyridoxal phosphate is reduced.

From all these facts and from our knowledge of the regulation of intracellular iron metabolism it follows that in the majority of sideroblastic anaemias a primary disorder of haem synthesis is of fundamental importance for the accumulation of non-haem iron in erythroblasts. Haem regulates the iron uptake by erythroid cells by limiting the release of iron from transferrin (*see* p. 45). If any enzyme of haem synthesis is inhibited, haem deficiency renders a more rapid dissociation of the iron-transferrin complex possible. Pathologic sideroblasts thus develop as a result of enhanced iron release from transferrin due to haem deficiency and not only by passive iron accumulation in cells caused by a reduced amount of protoporphyrin (*Poňka* and *Neuwirt*, 1974, 1975b). Iron released from transferrin accumulates in mitochondria as it cannot be utilized for haem synthesis (Fig. 57).

In some cases of sideroblastic anaemia iron accumulation is probably due to a primary disorder in the control of iron uptake by erythroid cells. It may be assumed that in this type of sideroblastic anaemia some disturbance of the cell membrane or intracellular iron transport is involved.

Excessive deposition of iron in the mitochondria of immature erythroid cells, whatever the primary cause, inhibits the activity of a number of enzymes, including · the enzymes of porphyrin metabolism. Thus a vicious circle develops because reduced porphyrin synthesis and reduced haem production further enhance iron dissociation from transferrin and excessive iron accumulation in mitochondria.

From the clinical aspect sideroblastic anaemias can be divided into hereditary forms with some inborn deficiency of haem synthesis, and acquired or secondary sideroblastic anaemias where haem synthesis is impaired by the toxic factors mentioned. Another clinical group are idiopathic sideroblastic anaemias which develop as a rule in the sixth decade. These idiopathic sideroblastic anaemias differ from other types by frequent association with neutropenia and thrombocytopenia. In idiopathic sideroblastic anaemias the iron containing granules are found in very primitive erythroid cells (Fig. 58) (*Hall* and *Losowsky*, 1966; *Wickramasinghe et al.*, 1971). Very often a megaloblastic transformation of the erythroid line is found without apparent folate deficiency and finally this form of sideroblastic anaemia very often changes into acute myeloid leukaemia (*Catovsky et al.*, 1971). Pathological sideroblasts are also sometimes observed in erythroleukaemia and in other forms of myelo-

170

proliferative diseases (*Dameshek*, 1965). The assumption has been submitted that these sideroblastic anaemias represent a certain entity in the large spectrum of myelo-proliferative diseases. It may be assumed that in this type of sideroblastic anaemias some hitherto not identified anomaly of the cell membrane of very immature erythroid precursors is involved. This disturbance of the cell membrane can be manifested on the one hand by increased iron penetration into immature cells and on the other it may play a part in the malignant transformation of these cells.

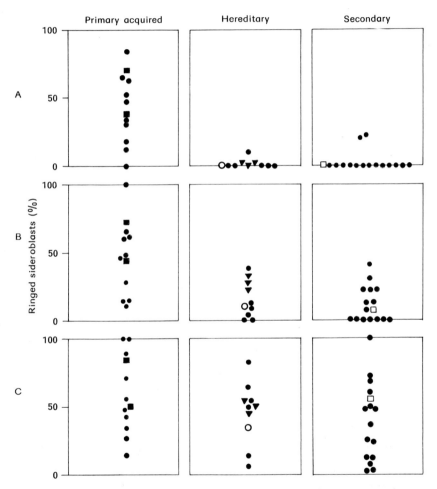

Fig. 58. Percentage of ringed sideroblasts in early (A), intermediate (B) and late (C) erythroblasts. Detailed description of patients with primary acquired (idiopathic), secondary and hereditary sideroblastic anaemias may be found in the original paper. Ringed sideroblasts rarely occur in early erythroblasts in the hereditary and secondary forms. (From *Hall* and *Losowsky*, 1966. Reproduced with the permission of the authors and the publisher.)

171

So far the cause of sideroblastic anaemias associated with rheumatoid arthritis, carcinomas, multiple myeloma, myxoedema, thyrotoxicosis, lymphoma, infectious mononucleosis and polyarthritis remains obscure. Sideroblastic anaemia is, however, extremely rare in these conditions.

HYPOCHROMIC ANAEMIAS DUE TO IMPAIRED GLOBIN SYNTHESIS

THALASSAEMIA

Thalassaemia is a heterogenoeous group of genetic disorders of haemoglobin synthesis which are characterized by an unbalanced production of globin chains. As a result of disorders of globin chain synthesis anaemia develops due to diminished haemoglobin formation and at the same time red cells in the periphery and bone marrow are destroyed in greater numbers. In the majority of thalassaemias pathological haemoglobin is not formed, although evidence is accumulating that some forms of thalassaemias are due to ineffective synthesis of globin chains with an abnormal structure.

Table 18

Haemoglobin synthesis in thalassaemia; development of technology for the elucidation of the molecular pathology

---

1. Relative rates of α- and ß-chain synthesis (*Weatherall et al.*, 1965; *Heywood et al.*, 1965; *Bank* and *Marks*, 1966).

2. Assembly time (translation and termination) of the α- and ß-chains (*Clegg et all.*, 1968; *Rieder*, 1972; *Clegg* and *Weatherall*, 1974).

3. Sizes of polysomes making α- and ß-chains as an estimate of chain initiation rate (*Nathan et al.*, 1971).

4. Isolation of mRNA and assay in cell-free system (*Nienhuis* and *Anderson*, 1971; *Benz* and *Forget*, 1971; *Benz et al.*, 1973; *Dow et al.*, 1973).

5. Estimation of total mRNA by cDNA/mRNA hybridization (*Housman et al.*, 1973; *Kacian et al.*, 1973).

6. Characterization of structure and synthesis of inefficiently produced structural haemoglobin variants:
   (a) Hb Lepore (*Baglioni*, 1962; *Roberts et al.*, 1972; *White et al.*, 1972);
   (b) α-chain termination mutants (*Clegg et al.*, 1971; *Weatherall* and *Clegg*, 1975b);
   (c) Hb K Woolwich (*Lang et al.*, 1974).

7. Determination of presence or absence of specific globin genes by cDNA/DNA hybridization (*Ottolenghi et al.*, 1974, 1975; *Taylor et al.*, 1974).

(From *Weatherall* and *Clegg*, 1975a. Reproduced with the permission of the authors and Blackwell Scientific Publications Ltd., Oxford.)

172

In recent years great advances have been made in the knowledge of the molecular pathology of thalassaemia (Table 18). It proved possible to isolate and assess human globin mRNA and moreover the method of cDNA/DNA hybridization for probing genetic fine structure was introduced.

In 1959 *Ingram* and *Stretton* divided thalassaemias into two large groups, α- and β-thalassaemias, depending on whether the synthesis of the α- or β-chain is affected. This basic classification still applies but it was revealed that many different types of α- and β-thalassaemias exist (*Weatherall* and *Clegg*, 1975). In particular forms of thalassaemia encountered in Asia and the Mediteranean area are well defined, while in Negro populations and in the Middle Eastern populations the mode of genetic transmission is not yet quite clear for some forms of thalassaemia.

α-thalassaemia

When the synthesis of α-chains is reduced or lacking, so-called α-thalassaemia develops. If there is a great reduction in the synthesis of α-chains, abnormal haemoglobin H formed by four normal β-chains is found in the cells (haemoglobin H disease). In the clinically most severe form of α-thalassaemia death in utero takes place (hydrops foetalis). α-chains are not synthesized at all and therefore no haemoglobin A is formed. As a result of a great excess of γ-chains Barts haemoglobin (γ_4) is formed as a foetal counterpart of haemoglobin H (Hb Barts hydrops syndrome). Barts haemoglobin as well as H-haemoglobin are useless from the functional aspect, as they bind oxygen but are unable to give it up to the tissues. Haemoglobin H is moreover unstable, precipitates and forms Heinz bodies. In contrast to β-thalassaemia, in the α-thalassaemia form haemoglobin A_2 or haemoglobin F are not elevated because the α-chains are part of both these haemoglobins.

It appears that Hb Barts hydrops syndrome and Hb H disease develop as a result of the interaction of three genes of α-thalassaemia, i.e. α-thal I, α-thal II and Hb Constant Spring. It has been proved that Hb Barts hydrops syndrome represents the homozygous state for the α-thal I gene. Haemoglobin H disease can develop from a heterozygous condition for both α-thal I and α-thal II genes or α-thal 0 and Hb Constant Spring form (*Wasi et al.*, 1974).

α- thalassaemia I. It has been already mentioned that subjects suffering from Hb Barts hydrops syndrome produce no α-chains. *Ottolenghi et al.* (1974) and *Taylor et al.* (1974) provided evidence that mRNA isolated from the liver of foetuses with Hb Barts hydrops syndrome in a cell-free system control only the synthesis of β- and γ-chains. When using hybridization techniques, unequivocal evidence was provided that genes for α-chains on the chromosomes of affected subjects are completely or almost completely lacking. This is the first case where it has been proved that gene deletion is the cause of a genetic disease in humans. At the same time these findings are evidence that α-thalassaemia I develops as a result of deletion of complete genes or the major part of genes for α-chains.

α-thalassaemia II. It has been proved that in some populations the human genes for α-genes are duplicated (*Lehmann* and *Lang*, 1974). It seems that α-thalassaemia II is caused by deletion of one of these genes similarly as α-thalassaemia I results from the loss of both genes. If this assumption is correct, Hb H disease develops in heterozygous subjects for α-thal I, where no α-chains are present and α-thal II, whereby only one functional locus for the α-chain remains. cDNA-RNA hybridization experiments provided evidence that in cells of patients with haemoglobin H disease the amount of mRNA for α-chains is reduced (*Housman et al.*, 1973). These findings showed that α-thalassaemia II develops as a result of deletion of one of the gene pairs for α-chains.

Haemoglobin Constant Spring and related mutants of the terminal portion of the chain

Hb Constant Spring is a haemoglobin with a prolonged α-chain with 31 added amino-acid residues at the C-terminal (*see* p. 121). The r;sidue in the 142 position is glutamine. This finding indicates that Hb Constant Spring develops by substitution of one base in the terminal codon. Normal UAA is replaced by CAA coding for glutamine. Instead of being terminated in position 141 the α-chain can grow until the next "stop" codon is reached.

So far it is not known why haemoglobin mutants of chain terminals are synthesized at a reduced rate. α-chains of Hb Constant Spring are synthesized actively only in nucleated red cells, while their synthesis has not been observed in reticulocytes. This indicates that mRNA for α-chains of Hb Constant Spring is relatively unstable.

There are a number of genetic phenomena suggesting that individuals who obtain α-thal I gene from one parent and the gene for Hb Constant Spring from the other parent have typical Hb H disease. This indicates that the Hb Constant Spring mutation behaves clinically exactly in the same way as the gene α-thal II.

β- and δβ-thalassaemia

It was revealed that this group of thalassaemias is also very heterogeneous from the genetic aspect. In the majority of so-called β+-thalassaemias a certain degree of synthesis of β-chains can always be found while in β°-thalassaemias the synthesis of the β-chain cannot be demonstrated.

In β+-thalassaemias the initiation, elongation and termination of the β-chain is quite normal (*Clegg et al.*, 1968; *Nathan et al.*, 1971). Assessment of total mRNA revealed that in β+-thalassaemia the activity of β-chain mRNA is reduced (*Nienhus* and *Anderson*, 1971; *Nienhus et al.*, 1973). cDNA/mRNA hybridization experiments provided evidence that the reduction of mRNA translation activity is due to a reduced amount of mRNA for β-chains (*Housman et al.*, 1973). From this ensues that β-thalassaemia develops as a result of reduced mRNA production, apparently because of impaired mRNA transcription and processing.

Synthesis of β-chains is not detectable in reticulocytes of patients with β°-thalassaemia. After addition to a cell-free system mRNA isolated from these reticulocytes is not capable of inducing synthesis of β-chains (*Dow et al.*, 1973). *Conconi et al.* (1972) described in Italy in the Ferrara area β°-thalassaemia where a certain amount of functional mRNA can be found. For an active β-chain synthesis, however, a soluble cellular fraction of normal reticulocytes must be added to the cell-free system. It cannot be ruled out that at least some cases of β°-thalassaemia are caused by synthesis of a very unstable mRNA for β-chains.

In δβ-thalassaemia there remain some obscure questions. Hb Lepore contains normal α-chains which combine with chains containing an N-terminal of δ-chains combined with C-terminal of β-chains. It seems that this disorder develops as a result of unequal crossing over between genes for δ- and β-chains with a resulting fusion of genes δβ, which then control the non-α-chain synthesis of Hb Lepore. It was found that in reticulocytes of individuals with Hb Lepore there is no detectable δβ-chain synthesis in reticulocytes, while their synthesis can be demonstrated in bone-marrow cells. This corresponds to the finding that synthesis of δ-chains during maturation declines considerably (*Rieder* and *Weatherhall*, 1965). *Clegg* and *Weatherhall* (1974) assumed that δ- and δβ-mRNA are unstable due to lack of sequences at the 5'- and 3'-ends of their mRNA. These sequences are present in α- and β-mRNA and act as stabilizing areas (*see* p. 101). It may be easily envisaged that degradation of such sensitive mRNA molecules can considerably reduce their levels in cells of subjects with the appropriate thalassaemia.

REFERENCES

Ackerman, G. A. (1962): Anat. Rec. 144, 239

Adamson S. D., Herbert E., Godchaux W. III (1968): Arch. Biochem. Biophys. *125*, 671

Adamson S. D., Herbert E., Kemp S. F. (1969a): J. mol. Biol. 42, 247

Adamson S. D., Howard G. A., Herbert E. (1969b): Cold Spring Harb. Symp. Quant. Biol. *34*, 547

Adamson S. D., Mo-Ping Yau P., Herbert E. (1972): J. mol. Biol. *63*, 247

Addison G. M., Beamish M. R., Hales C. N., Hodkins M., Jacobs A., Llewellin P. (1972): J. clin. Pathol. *25*, 326

Aisen P., Leibman A. (1968): Biochem. biophys. Res. Commun. 32, 220

Aisen P., Leibman A. (1973): Biochim. biophys. Acta *304*, 797

Alfrey C. P., Lynch E. C., Whitley C. E. (1967): J. Lab. clin. Med. *70*, 419

Allen D. W. (1960): Blood *16*, 1564

Allen D. W., Jandl J. H. (1960): Blood *15*, 71

Allen E. H., Schweet R. S. (1962): J. biol. Chem. *237*, 760

Alpen E. L., Cranmore D. (1959): Ann. N.Y. Acad. Sci. *77*, 753

Anderson W. F. (1972) In: Synthesis, Structure and Function of Haemoglobin (Ed. by Martin, H. and Nowicki, L.), Lehmanns Verlag, München, p. 109

Anderson W. F. (1974): Ann. N.Y. Acad. Sci. *232*, 15

Anderson W. F., Barker J. E., Elson N. A., Merrick W. C., Steggles A. W., Wilson G. N., Kantor J. A., Nienhuis A. W. (1975): J. cell. Physiol. *85*, 477

Anderson W. F., Shafritz D. A. (1971): Cancer Res. *31*, 701

Antonioli J. A., Christensen H. N. (1969): J. biol. Chem. *244*, 1505

Aoki Y., Urata G., Wada O. (1974): J. clin. Invest. *53*, 1326

Aoki Y., Wada O., Urata G., Takaku F., Nakao K. (1971): Biochem. biophys. Res. Commun. *42*, 568

Appleton T. C., Morgan E. H., Baker E. (1971) In: The Regulation of Erythropoiesis and Haemoglobin Synthesis. (Ed. by Trávníček T. and Neuwirt J.), Universita Karlova, Praha, p. 310

Arlinghaus R., Favelukes G., Schweet R. (1963): Biochem. biophys. Res. Commun. *11*, 92

Arlinghaus R., Schaeffer J., Bishop J., Schweet R. (1968): Arch. Biochem. Biophys. *125*, 604

Arlinghaus R., Schaeffer J., Schweet R. (1964): Proc. nat. Acad. Sci. (Wash.): *51*, 1291

Arnstein H. R. V., Cox R. A., Gould H., Potter H. (1965): Biochem. J. *96*, 500

Aviv H., Boime I., Leder P. (1971): Proc. nat. Acad. Sci. (Wash.) *68*, 2303

Axel R., Cedar H., Felsenfeld G. (1973): Proc. nat. Acad. Sci. (Wash.) *70*, 2029

Axelrad A. A., McLeod D. L., Shreeve M. M., Heath D. S. (1974): Properties of cells that produce erythrocytic colonies in vitro. In: Hemopoiesis in Culture, Second International Workshop (Ed. by Robinson W. A.), U.S. Government Printing Office, Washington, p. 226

Bachvaroff R. J., Tongur V. (1966): Nature (Lond.) *211*, 248

Baglioni C. (1962): Proc. nat. Acad. Sci. (Wash.) *48*, 1880

Baglioni C., Campana T. (1967): Europ. J. Biochem. *2*, 480

Bainton D. F., Finch C. A. (1964): Amer. J. Med. *1*, 62

Baker E., Morgan E. H. (1969a): Biochemistry *8*, 1133

Baker E., Morgan E. H. (1969b): Biochemistry *8*, 2954

176

Baker E., Morgan E. H. (1971): J. cell. Physiol. 77, 377

Balkow K., Hunt T., Jackson R. J. (1975): Biochem. biophys. Res. Commun. 67, 366

Balkow K., Mizuno S., Fisher J. M., Rabinovitz M. (1973a): Biochim. biophys. Acta (Amst.) 324, 397

Balkow K., Mizuno S., Rabinovitz M. (1973b); Biochim. biophys. Acta (Amst.) 54, 315

Bank A., Braverman A. S., O'Donnell J. V., Marks P. A. (1968): Blood 31, 226

Bank A., Marks P. A. (1966): Nature (Lond.) 212, 1198

Bank A., Marks P. A. (1969): Med. Clin. N. Amer. 53, 875

Bank A., O'Donnell J. V. (1969): Nature (Lond.) 222, 295

Barnes R., Connelly J. L., Jones O. T. G. (1972): Biochem. J. 128, 1043

Barnett H. LaDona, Archdeacon J. W. (1970): Biochim. biophys. Acta (Amst.) 219, 231

Bates G. W., Schlabach M. R. (1973): FEBS Letters 33, 289

Bates G. W., Schlabach M. R. (1975): In: Proteins of Iron Storage and Transport in Biochemistry and Medicine (Ed. by Crichton, R. R.) North-Holland Publishing Company, Amsterdam, p. 51

Beard N. S., Jr., Armentrout S. A., Weisberger A. S. (1969): Pharmacol. Rev. 21, 213–245

Beaudet A. L., Caskey C. T. (1971): Proc. nat. Acad. Sci. (Wash.) 68, 619

Beaudet A. L., Caskey C. T. (1971): Proc. nat. Acad. Sci. (Wash.) 68, 619

Beck E. A., Ziegler G., Schmid R. (1967): Acta haemat. (Basel) 38, 1

Bedard D. L., Goldwasser E. (1976): Exp. Cell Res. 102, 376

Belcher E. H., Courtenay V. D. (1959): Brit. J. Haemat. 5, 268

Benz E. J., Jr., Forget B. G. (1971): J. clin. Invest. 50, 2755

Benz E. J., Jr., Forget B. G. (1974): Semin. Hemat. 11, 463

Benz E., Swerdlow P. S., Forget B. G. (1973): Blood 42, 825

Bessis, M. C. (1963): Harvey Lect. Ser. 58, 125

Bessis M. C., Breton-Gorius J. (1959): Blood 14, 423

Bessis M. C., Breton-Gorius J. (1962): Blood 19, 635

Bessis M. C., Jensen W. N. (1965): Brit. J. Haemat. 11, 49

Beuzard Y., London I. M. (1974): Proc. nat. Acad. Sci. (Wash.) 71, 2863–2866

Beuzard Y., Rodvien R., London I. M. (1973): Proc. nat. Acad. Sci. (Wash.) 70, 1022

Bezkorovainy A., Zschmocke R. H. (1974): Arzneimittel-Forsch. 24, 476

Bhaduri S., Chatterjee N. K., Bose K. K., Gupta N. K. (1970): Biochem. biophys. Res. Commun. 40, 402

Biehl J. P., Vilter R. W. (1954): J. Amer. med. Ass. 156, 1549

Bishop J. O. (1965): Nature (Lond.) 208, 361

Bishop J. O. (1966a): Biochim. biophys. Acta (Amst.) 119, 130

Bishop J. O. (1966b): J. mol. Biol. 17, 285

Bishop J., Favelukes G., Schweet R., Russel E. (1961): Nature (Lond.) 191, 1365

Bishop J. O., Pemberton R. E., Baglioni C. (1972): Nature New Biol. 235, 231

Bishop J. O., Rosbach M. (1973): Nature New Biol. 241, 204

Blackburn G. W., Morgan E. H. (1976): Biochim. biophys. Acta (Amst.) (in press)

Blobel G. (1971): Proc. nat. Acad. Sci. (Wash.) 68, 832

Blobel G. (1972): Biochem. biophys. Res. Commun. 47, 88

Blum N., Kneip B., Schapira G. (1972): Biochimie 54, 1121

Blum N., Maleknia N., Schapira G. (1969): Biochim. biophys. Acta (Amst.) *179*, 448
Blum N., Maleknia M., Schapira G. (1970): Biochim. biophys. Acta (Amst.) *199*, 236
Blum N., Schapira G. (1967): C.R. Acad. Sci (D) *264*, 1211
Bonanou S. A., Arnstein H. R. V. (1969): FEBS Letters *3*, 348
Bonanou-Tzedaki S. A., Pragnell I. B., Arnstein H. R. V. (1972): FEBS Letters *26*, 77
Booij H. L., Rimington C. (1957): Biochem. J. *65*, 4P
Borová J., Fuchs O., Poňka P., Neuwirt J. (1976): Collection Czechoslov. Chem. Commun. *41*, 2448
Borová J., Poňka P., Neuwirt J. (1973): Biochim. biophys. Acta (Amst.) *320*, 143
Borsook H. (1964): Blood *24*, 202
Borsook H., Lingrel J. B., Scaro J. L., Milette R. L. (1962): Nature (Lond.) *196*, 347
Borsook H., Ratner K., Tattrie B., Teigler D., Lajtha L. G. (1968a): Nature (Lond.) *217*, 1024
Borsook H., Teigler D., Gunderson A. (1968b): Arch. Biochem. Biophys. *125*, 429
Bothwell T. H., Finch C. A. (1962) In: Iron Metabolism, Little, Brown and Co., Boston
Bottomley S. S. (1968): Blood *31*, 322
Bottomley S. S., Smithee G. A. (1968): Biochim. biophys. Acta (Amst.) *159*, 27
Bottomley S. S., Smithee G. A. (1969): Blood *34*, 857
Bottomley S. S., Smithee G. A. (1969b): J. Lab. clin. Med. *74*, 445
Bottomley S. S., Whitcomb W. H., Smithee G. A., Moore M. Z. (1971): J. Lab. clin. Med. *77*, 793
Boyer S. H., Smith D. K., Noyes N. A., Mullen M. A. (1974): J. biol. Chem. *249*, 7210
Brawerman G., Biezunski N., Eisenstadt J. (1965): Biochim. biophys. Acta (Amst.) *103*, 201
Brecher G., Stohlman F. Jr. (1962) In: Erythropoiesis (Ed. by L. O. Jacobson and M. Doyle). Grune and Stratton, New York, p. 216
Brecher G., Stohlman F. (1961): Proc. Soc. exp. Biol. Med. *107*, 887
Brenner S., Jacob F., Meselson M. (1961): Nature (Lond.) *190*, 576
Brown E. B. (1975) In: Proteins of Iron Storage and Transport in Biochemistry and Medicine (Ed. by Crichton, R. R.) North Holland Publishing Company, Amsterdam, p. 97
Brown E. G. (1958): Biochem. J. *70*, 313
Brown J. E., Adamson J. W. (1974): Blood *44*, 913
Bruce W. R., McCulloch E. A. (1964): Blood *23*, 216
Bruns G. P., London I. M. (1965): Biochem. biophys. Res. Commun. *18*, 236
Bulova S. I., Burka E. R. (1970): J. biol. Chem. *245*, 4907
Bunn H. F., Jandl J. H. (1968): J. biol. Chem. *243*, 465
Bunn H. F., Schmidt G. J., Dluhy R. G. (1975): Proc. nat. Acad. Sci. (Wash.) 72, 3609
Burka E. R. (1968): Science *162*, 1287
Burka E. R., Schreml W., Kick C.: Biochem. biophys. Res. Commun. *26*, 334–338
Burka E. R., Schreml W., Kick C. J. (1967b): Biochemistry *6*, 2840
Burke G. T., Goldstein J., Redman G. M. (1973): FEBS Letters *37*, 221
Burnham B. F. (1963): Acta chem. Scand. *17*, 123
Burnham B. F., Lascelles J. (1963): Biochem. J. *87*, 462
Burr H., Lingrel J. B. (1971): Nature New Biol. *233*, 41
Byrnes J. J., Downey K. M., Jurmark, B. S. (1974): Nature (Lond.) *248*, 687
Byrnes J. J., Downey K. M., Esserman L., So A. G. (1975): Biochemistry *14*, 796

Cahn F., Lubin M. (1975): Mol. Biol. Rep. *2*, 49

Calissano P., Bonsignore D., Cartesegna C. (1966): Biochem. J. *101*, 550

Cann A. A., Gambino R., Banks J., Bank A. (1974): J. biol. Chem. *249*, 7536

Cantor L. N., Morris A. J., Marks P. A., Rifkind R. A. (1972): Proc. nat. Acad. Sci (Wash.)
69, 1337

Čáp J., Lehotská V., Mayerová A. (1968): Čs. Pediat. *23*, 1020

Cartwright G. E., Deiss A. (1975): New Engl. J. Med. *292*, 185

Cartwright G. E., Gubler C. J., Bush J. A., Wintrobe M. M. (1956): Blood *11*, 43

Cashion L. M., Stanley W. M. (1974): Proc. nat. Acad. Sci. (Wash.) *71*, 436

Catovsky D., Shaw M. T., Hoffbrand A. V. (1971): Brit. J. Haemat. *20*, 385

Chang C.-S., Goldwasser E. (1973): Develop. Biol. *34*, 246

Chang S. C.-S., Sikkema D., Goldwasser E. (1974): Biochem. biophys. Res. Commun. *57*, 399

Chantrenne H., Burny A., Marbaix G. (1967): Progr. Nucleic Acid Res. mol. Biol. *7*, 173

Chen Y. C., Woodley C. L., Bose K. K., Gupta N. K. (1972): Biochem. biophys. Res. Commun.
48, 1

Cheng T., Polmar S. K., Kazazian H. H., Jr. (1974): J. Biol. Chem. *249*, 1781

Chernelch M., Brown E. B. (1970): Nature (Lond.) *226*, 356

Christman J. K., Goldstein J. (1969): Biochim. biophys. Acta (Amst.) *179*, 280

Chui D. H. K., Djaldetti M., Marks P. A., Rifkind R. A. (1971): J. cell. Biol. *51*, 585

Clark B. F. C., Marcker K. A. (1965): Nature (Lond.) *207*, 1038

Clark B. F. C., Marcker K. A. (1966): J. mol. Biol. *17*, 394

Clark P., Walsh R. J. (1959): Nature (Lond.) *184*, 1731

Clark P., Walsh R. J. (1960): Aust. J. exp. Biol. med. Sci. *38*, 135

Clegg J. B. (1974): Clinics in Haematol. *3*, 225

Clegg J. B., Naughton M. A., Weatherall D. J. (1965): Nature (Lond.) *207*, 945

Clegg J. B., Weatherall D. J. (1974): Ann. N.Y. Acad. Sci *232*, 168

Clegg J. B., Weatherall D. J. (1974): Lancet *ii*, 133

Clegg J. B., Weatherall D. J., Eunson C. E. (1971a): Biochim. biophys. Acta (Amst.) *247*, 109

Clegg J. B., Weatherall D. J., Milner P. F. (1971b): Nature (Lond.) *234*, 337

Clegg J. B., Weatherall D. J., Na-Nakorn S., Wasi P. (1968): Nature (Lond.) *220*, 664

Clemens M. J., Henshaw E. C., Rahamimoff H., London I. M. (1974): Proc. nat. Acad. Sci. (Wash.)
71, 2946

Clemens M. J., Safer B., Merrick W. C., Anderson W. F., London I. M. (1975): Proc. nat. Acad.
Sci. (Wash.) *72*, 1286

Cleton F., Turnbull A., Finch C. A. (1963): J. clin. Invest. *42*, 327

Cohen B. B. (1969): Biochem. J. *115*, 523

Cohen B. B. (1970): FEBS Letters *6*, 61

Cohen B. B. (1971): Biochim. biophys. Acta (Amst.) *247*, 133

Colombo B., Baglioni C. (1966): J. mol. Biol. *16*, 51

Colombo B., Vesco C., Baglioni C. (1968): Proc. nat. Acad. Sci. (Wash.) *61*, 651

Conconi F., Rowley P. T., del Senno L., Pontremoli S. (1972): Nature New Biol. *238*, 83

Congote L. F., Stern M. D., Solomon S. (1974): Biochemistry *13*, 4255

Conkie D., Kleiman C., Harrison P. P., Paul J. (1975): Exp. cell. Res. *93*, 315

Cooper R. G., Webster L. T., Jr., Harris J. W. (1963): J. clin. Invest. *42*, 926

Coutelle C., Ryskov A. P., Georgiev G. P. (1970): FEBS Letters *12*, 21

Cox R. A., Arnstein H. R. V. (1963): Biochem. J. *89*, 574

Cox R. A., Bonanou S. A. (1969): Biochem. J. *114*, 769

Crystal R. G., Nienhuis A. W., Elson N. A., Anderson W. F. (1972): J. biol. Chem. *247*, 5357

Crystal R. G., Shafritz D. A., Prichard P. M., Anderson W. F. (1971): Proc. nat. Acad. Sci. (Wash.) *68*, 1810

Dabney B. J., Beaudet A. L. (1976): Fed. Proc. 35, 1976

Dagg J. H., Goldberg A., Lochead A., Smith J. A. (1965): Quart. J. Med. *34*, 163

Dallman P. R., Loskutoff D. (1967): J. clin. Invest. *46*, 1819

Dameshek W. (1965): Brit. J. Haemat. *11*, 52

Datta M. C., Dukes P. P. *(1975)*: Biochem. biophys. Res. Commun. *66*, 293

Darnbrough C., Hunt T., Jackson R. (1972): Biochem. biophys. Res. Commun. *48*, 1556

Darnbrough C., Legon S., Hunt T., Jackson R. J. (1973): J. mol. Biol. *76*, 379

Darnell J. E., Jelinek W. R., Molloy G. R. (1973): Science *181*, 1215

Davidson E. H., Britten R. J. (1973): Quart. Rev. Biol. *48*, 565

Davis B. D. (1971): Nature (Lond.) *231*, 153

Debellis R. H., Gluck N., Marks P. A. (1964): J. clin. Invest. *43/7*, 1329

Deiss A., Cartwright G. E. (1970): J. clin. Invest. *49*, 517

Del Monte M. A., Kazazian H. H. Jr. (1971): J. mol. Biol. *56*, 429

Dibble W. E., Dintzis H. M. (1960): Biochim. biophys. Acta (Amst.) *37*, 152

Dintzis H. M. (1961): Proc. nat. Acad. Sci. (Wash.) *47*, 247

Dintzis H. M., Borsook H., Vinograd J. (1958) In: Microsomal Particles and Protein Synthesis (Ed. by Roberts, R. B.) Pergamon Press Ltd London, p. 95

Djaldetti M., Preisler H. S., Marks P. A., Rifkind R. A. (1972): J. biol. Chem. *247*, 731

Dow L. W., Terada M., Natta C., Metafora S., Grossbard E., Marks P. A., Bank A. (1973): Nature New Biol. *243*, 114

Downey K. M., Byrnes J. J., Jurmark B. S., So A. G. (1973): Proc. nat. Acad. Sci. (Wash.) *70*, 3400

Drach J. C., Lingrel J. B. (1964): Biochem biophys. Acta (Amst.) *91*, 680

Drach J. C., Lingrel J. B. (1966): Biochim. biophys. Acta (Amst.) *123*, 345

Drach J. C., Lingrel J. B. (1966b): Biochim. biophys. Acta (Amst.) *129*, 178

Dresel E. I. B., Falk I. E. (1956): Biochem. J. *63*, 72

Dukes P. P. (1968): Ann. N.Y. Acad. Sci 149/Art. *1*, 437

Dukes P. P. (1968b): Biochem. biophys. Res. Commun. *31*, 345

Dukes P. P., Takaku F., Goldwasser E. (1964): Endocrinology *74*, 960

DuVigneaud V., Kuckinskas E. J., Horvath A. (1957): Arch. Biochem. Biophys. *69*, 130

Ebert P. S., Ikawa Y. (1974): Proc. Soc. exp. Biol. (N.Y.) *146*, 601

Edwards J. A. (1970): Biochim. biophys. Acta (Amst.) *204*, 280

Edwards S. A., Fielding J. (1971): Brit. J. Haemat. *20*, 405

Efron D., Marcus A. (1973): FEBS Letters *33*, 23

Egyed A. (1973): Biochim. biophys. Acta (Amst.) *304*, 805

Egyed A. (1974): Acta Biochim. Biophys. Acad. Sci. Hung. *9*, 43

Ehrenfeld E., Hunt T. (1971): Proc. nat. Acad. Sci (Wash.) *68*, 1075

Eichner E. R., Hillman R. S. (1971): Amer. J. Med. *50*, 218

Eldor A., Manny N., Izak G. (1970): Blood *36*, 233

Ernst V., Arnstein H. R. V. (1975): Biochim. biophys. Acta (Amst.) *378*, 251

Ernst V., Levin D. H., Ranu R. S., London I. M. (1976): Proc. nat. Acad. Sci. (Wash.) *73*, 1112

Erslev A. J., Hughes J. R. (1960): Brit. J. Haemat. *6*, 414

Erslev A. J., Iossifides I. A. (1962): Acta haemat. (Basel) *28*, 1

Eylar E. H., Matioli G. (1965): Nature (Lond.) *208*, 661

Falbe-Hansen I., Lothe K. (1962): Acta physiol. Scand. *54*, 97

Falk J. E., Porra R. J., Brown A., Moss F., Larminie H. E. (1959): Nature (Lond.) *184/4694*, 1217

Feinendegen L. E., Bond V. P., Cronkite E. P., Hughes W. L. (1964): Ann. N.Y. Acad. Sci. *113*, 727

Falvey A. K., Staehelin T. (1970): J. mol. Biol. 53, 1

Fantoni A., ae la Chapelle A., Rifkind R. A., Marks P. A. (1968): J. mol. Biol. *33*, 79

Feeney R. E., Allison R. G. (1969): Evolutionary Biochemistry of Proteins. Wiley-Interscience, New York, London, Sydney and Toronto

Feldman I'., Lightman H. C. (1967): Biochim. biophys. Acta (Amst.) *141*, 653

Felicetti L., Colombo B., Baglioni, C. (1966): Biochim. biophys. Acta (Amst.) *129*, 380

Fessas P., Loukopoulos D. (1964): Science *143*, 590

Fielding J., Edwards S. A., Ryall R. (1969): J. clin. Pathol. *22*, 677

Fielding J., Speyer B. E. (1974): Biochim. biophys. Acta (Amst.) *363*, 387

Filipowicz W., Sierra J. M., Nombela C., Ochoa S., Merrick W. C., Anderson W. F. (1976): Proc. nat. Acad. Sci. (Wash.) *73*, 44

Finch C. A. (1969): Amer. J. clin. Nutr. *22*, 512

Finch C. A. (1970): Diagnostic value of different methods to detect iron deficiency. In: Iron Deficiency. (Eds. Hallberg L., Harwerth H. G. and Vannotti A.) Academic Press, London and New York, p. 409

Fletcher J., Huehns E. R. (1967): Nature (Lond.) 215, 584

Fletcher J., Huehns E. R. (1968): Nature (Lond.) 218, 1211

Forget B. G., Benz E. J., Jr. (1974): Nature (Lond.) 247, 379

Forget B. G., Benz E. J., Jr., Skoultchi A., Baglioni C., Housman D. (1974): Nature (Lond.) 247, 379

Forget B. G., Marotta C. A., Weissman S., Cohen-Solal M. (1975): Proc. nat. Acad. Sci (Wash.) 72(9), 3614

Forte F. J., Cohen H. S., Rosman J., Freedman M. L. (1976): Blood *47*, 145

Freedman M. L., Cohen H. S., Rosman J., Forte F. J. (1975): Brit. J. Haemat. *30*, 351

Freedman M. L., Honig G. R., Rabinovitz M. (1966): Exp. Cell Res. *44*, 263

Freedman M. L., Rabinovitz M. (1970): Exp. Cell Res. *60*, 480

Freedman M. L., Rosman J. (1976): J. clin. Invest. 57, 1976

Friend C. (1957): J. exp. Med. *105*, 307

Friend C., Patuleia M. C., De Harven E. (1966): Nat. Cancer Inst. Monograph *22*, 505

Friend C., Scherr W., Holland J. H., Sato T. (1971): Proc. nat. Acad. Sci (Wash.) *68*, 378

Frydman R. B., Tomaro M. L., Wanschelbaum A., Frydman B. (1973): Enzyme *16*, 160

Frydman R. B., Valasinas A., Frydman B. (1973): Enzyme *16*, 151

Fuchs O., Borová J., Poňka P., Neuwirt J. (1976): Biochem. clin. Bohemoslov. *7*, 161

Fuchs O., Borová J., Poňka P., Neuwirt J., Nečas E. (1975): Proc. of the 2nd International Congress on Pathological Physiology, Prague (Abstr. No. 105)

181

Fuhr J. E., Gengozian N. (1973): Biochim. biophys. Acta (Amst.) *320*, 53

Fuhr J., Natta C. (1972): Nature New Biol. *240*, 274

Fuhr J. E., Natta C., Bank A., Marks P. A. (1971): Biochim. biophys. Acta (Amst.) *240*, 70

Gabuzda T. G., Gardner F. H. (1967): Blood *29*, 770

Gabuzda T. G., Pearson J. (1968): Nature (Lond.) *220*, 1234

Gabuzda T. G., Pearson J. (1969): Biochim. biophys. Acta (Amst.) *194*, 50

Gajdos A., Gajdos-Török M. (1969): Biochem. Med. *2*, 372

Gajdos A., Gajdos-Török M. (1973): Enzyme *16*, 101

Galizzi A. (1969): Europ. J. Biochem. *10*, 561

Gallo R. C. (1967): J. clin. Invest. *46*, 124

Gambino R., Kacian D., O'Donnell J., Ramirez F., Marks P. A., Bank A. (1974): Proc. nat. Acad. Sci. (Wash.) *71*, 3966

Ganzoni A. M. (1968): Helv. med. Acta *34*, 416

Ganzoni A. M., Hahn D., Späti B. (1972): Blut *24*, 269

Garrett N. E., Garrett R. J. B., Archdeacon J. W. (1973): Biochim. biophys. Res. Commun. *52*, 466

Garrick L. M., Dembuke P. P., Garrick M. D. (1975): Europ. J. Biochem. 58, 339

Gaskill P., Kabat O. (1971): Proc. nat. Acad. Sci. (Wash.) *68*, 72

Gazaryan K. G., Tarantul V. Z., Barranov Yu. N., Frolova L. Yu., Kiselev L. L. (1974): Dokl. Akad. Nauk SSSR *216*, 216

George W. J., Rodgers G. M., Briggs D. W., Fisher J. W. (1975) In: Erythropoiesis. Proceedings of the Fourth International Conference on Erythropoiesis (Ed. by Nakao K., Fisher J. W. and Takaku F.). University of Tokyo Press, p. 277

Georgiev G. P. (1962): Biochim. biophys. Acta (Amst.) *61*, 153

Georgiev G. P., Ryskov A. P., Coutelle C., Mantieva V. L., Avakyan E. R. (1972): Biochim. biophys. Acta (Amst.) *259*, 259

Georgiev G. P., Samatina O. P., Lerman M. L., Smirnov M. N., Severtzov A. N. (1963): Nature (Lond.) *200*, 1291

Gianni A. M., Giglioni B., Ottolenghi S., Comi P., Guidotti G. G. (1972): Nature New Biol. *240*, 183

Gibson K. D. (1955) In: Ciba Fdn. Symp. on Porphyrin Biosynthesis and Metabolism. (Ed. by G. E. W. Wolstenholme and E. C. P. Millar), J. & A. Churchill Ltd., London, p. 27

Gibson K. D., Laver W. G., Neuberger A. (1958): Biochem. J. *70*, 71

Gibson K. D., Matthew M., Neuberger A., Tait G. H. (1961): Nature (Lond.) *192*, 204

Gierer A. (1963): J. mol. Biol. *6*, 148

Giglioni B., Gianni A. M., Comi P., Ottolenghi S., Rungger D. (1973): Nature New Biol. (1973): *246*, 99

Gilbert J. M., Anderson W. F. (1970): J. biol. Chem. *245*, 2342

Gilmour R. S. (1973): Nature (Lond.) *246*, 8

Gilmour R. S., Harrison P. R., Windass J. D., Affara N. A., Paul J. (1974): Cell Differentiation *3*, 9

Gilmour R. S., Paul J. (1973): Proc. nat. Acad. Sci (Wash.) *70*, 3440

Gilmour R. S., Windass J. D., Affara N., Paul J. (1975): J. cell. Physiol. *85*, 449

Glass J., Lavidor L. M., Robinson S. H. (1975a): J. cell. Biol. *65*, 298

Glass J., Yannoni C. Z., Robinson S. H. (1975b): Blood Cells *1*, 557

182

Glišin V., Crkvenjakov R., Byus C. (1974): Biochemistry *13*, 2633

Godchaux, W. III, Adamson S. D., Herbert E. (1967): J. mol. Biol. *27*, 57

Godin C., Kruh J., Dreyfus J. C. (1969): Biochim. biophys. Acta (Amst.) *182*, 175

Goldberg A., Aschenbrucker H., Cartwright G. E., Wintrobe M. M. (1956): Blood *11*, 821

Goldstein J. L., Beaudet A. L., Caskey C. T. (1970): Proc. nat. Acad. Sci. (Wash.) *67*, 99

Goldwasser E. (1975a) In: Erythropoiesis. Proceedings of the Fourth International Conference on Erythropoiesis (Ed. by Nakao K., Fisher J. W. and Takaku F.), University of Tokyo Press, p. 75

Goldwasser E. (1975b): Feder. Proc. *34*, 2285

Gonano F., Baglioni C. (1969): Europ. J. Biochem. *11*, 7

Goodman H. M., Rich A. (1963): Nature (Lond.) *199*, 318

Goodman J. R., Dallman P. R. (1969): Blood *34*, 747

Goodman J. R., Hall S. G. (1967): Brit. J. Haemat. *13*, 335

Gorski J., Morrison M. R., Merkel C. G., Lingrel J. B. (1974): J. mol. Biol. *86*, 363

Goucher C. R., Taylor J. F. (1964): J. biol. Chem. *239*, 2251

Gould H. J., Arnstein H. R. V., Cox R. A. (1966): J. mol. Biol. *15*, 600

Gould H. J., Hamlyn P. H. (1973): FEBS Letters *30*, 301

Goya N., Miyazaki S., Kodate S., Ushino B. (1972): Blood *40*, 239

Graber S. E., Carrillo M., Krantz S. B. (1972): Proc. Soc. exp. Biol. (N.Y.) *141*, 206

Graber S. E., Carrillo M., Krantz S. B. (1974): J. Lab. clin. Med. *83*, 288

Granick S. (1958): J. biol. Chem. *232*, 1101

Granick S. (1966): J. biol. Chem. *241*, 1359

Granick S., Kappas A. (1967): Proc. nat. Acad. Sci. (Wash.) *57*, 1463

Granick S., Lvere E. D. (1964) In: Progress in Hematology. (Ed. by C. V. Moore and E. B. Brown.) Grune and Stratton, New York, vol. 4, p. 1

Granick S., Mauzerall D. (1958): Ann. N.Y. Acad. Sci. *75*, 115

Granick S., Sano S. (1961): Fed. Proc. *20/1*, 376

Granick S., Urata G. (1963): J. biol. Chem. *238*, 821

Grasso J. A., Hines J. D. (1969): Brit. J. Haemat. *17*, 35

Grasso J. A., Woodard J. W. (1966): J. Cell Biol. *31*, 279

Grasso J. A., Woodard J. W. (1967): J. Cell Biol. *33*, 645

Grasso J. A., Woodard J. W., Swift R. (1963): Proc. nat. Acad. Sci. (Wash.) *50*, 134

Grayzel A. I., Fuhr J. E., London I. M. (1967): Biochim. biophys. Res. Commun. *28*, 705

Grayzel A. I., Hörchner P., London I. M. (1966): Proc. nat. Acad. Sci (Wash.) *55*, 650

Greenough, W. B., Peters T. Jr., Thomas E. D. (1962): J. clin. Invest. *41*, 1116

Grollman A. P. (1966): Proc. nat. Acad. Sci. (Wash.) *56*, 1867

Grollman A. P. (1968): J. biol. Chem. *243*, 4089

Gross M. (1974a): Biochim. biophys. Acta (Amst.) *340*, 484

Gross M. (1974b): Biochim. biophys. Acta (Amst.) *366*, 319

Gross M. (1975): Biochem. biophys. Res. Commun. *67*, 1507

Gross M., Goldwasser E. (1968): Fed. Proc. *27*, 394

Gross M., Goldwasser E. (1969): Biochemistry *8*, 1795

Gross M., Goldwasser E. (1970): J. biol. Chem. *245*, 1632

Gross M., Goldwasser E. (1971): J. biol. Chem. *246*, 2480

Gross M., Goldwasser E. (1972): Biochim. biophys. Acta (Amst.) 287, 514

Gross M., Rabinovitz M. (1972a): Biochim. biophys. Acta (Amst.) 287, 340

Gross M., Rabinovitz M. (1972b): Proc. nat. Acad. Sci. (Wash.) 69, 1565

Gross M., Rabinovitz M. (1973a): Biochem. biophys. Res. Commun. 50, 832

Gross M., Rabinovitz M. (1973b): Biochim. biophys. Acta (Amst.) 299, 472

Gummerson K. S., Williamson R. (1974): Nature (Lond.) 247, 265

Gupta N. K., Aerni R. J. (1973): Biochem. biophys. Res. Commun. 51, 907

Gupta N. K., Chatterjee N. K., Bose K. K., Bhaduri S., Chung A. (1970): J. mol. Biol. 54, 145

Gupta N. K., Chatterjee B., Chen Y. C., Majmudar A. (1974): Biochem. biophys. Res. Commun. 58, 699

Gupta N. K., Chatterjee N. K., Woodley C. L., Bose K. K. (1971): J. biol. Chem. 246, 7460

Gupta N. K., Woodley C. L., Chen Y. C., Bose K. K. (1973): J. biol. Chem. 248, 4500

Gurdon J. B. (1973): Acta endocrin. 74 (Suppl. 180), 225

Gurdon J. B., Lane C. D., Woodland H. R., Marbaix G. (1971): Nature (Lond.) 233, 177

Gurdon J. B., Lingrel J. B., Marbaix G. (1973): J. mol. Biol. 80, 539

Gurdon J. B., Woodland H. R., Lingrel J. B. (1974): Develop. Biol. 39, 125

Gurney C. W., Lajtha L. G., Oliver R. (1962): Brit. J. Haemat. 8, 461

Hahn D. (1973): Europ. J. Biochem. 34, 311

Hall N. D., Arnstein H. R. V. (1973): FEBS Letters 35, 45

Hall R., Losowsky M. S. (1966): Brit. J. Haemat. 12, 334

Hamada K., Yang P., Heintz R., Schweet R. (1968): Arch. Biochem. Biophys. 125, 598

Hammel C. L., Bessman S. P. (1964): J. biol. Chem. 239, 2228

Hardesty B., Culp W., McKeehan W. (1969): Cold Spring Harb. Symp. Quant. Biol. 34, 331

Hardesty B., Culp W., Odom O. W., Oliver R. M. (1972) In: Synthesis, Structure and Function of Haemoglobin. (Ed. by Martin H. and Nowicki L.) Lehmanns Verlag, München, p. 147

Harris D. C., Aisen P. (1975): Biochemistry 14, 262

Harriss E. B., MacGibbon B. H., Mollin D. L. (1965): Brit. J. Haemat. 11, 99

Harris H. (1967): J. Cell. Sci. 2, 23

Harris J. W. (1964): Medicine 43, 803

Harrison P. H. (1964) In: Iron Metabolism. (Ed. by F. Gross). Berlin, Springer Verlag, p. 40

Harrison P. R., Conkie D., Paul J., Jones K. (1973): FEBS Letters 32, 109

Harrison P. R., Gilmour R. S., Affara N. A., Conkie D., Paul J. (1974): Cell Differentiation 3, 23

Harrison P. R., Hell A., Birnie G. D., Paul J. (1972): Nature (Lond.) 239, 219

Haselkorn R., Rothman-Denes L. B. (1973): Ann. Rev. Biochem. 42, 397

Haurani F., Burke W., Martinez E. J. (1965): J. Lab. clin. Med. 65, 560

Haut M. S., Kark J. A., McQuilkin C. T., Gibson T. P., Hicks C. U. (1975): Abstr. International Soc. of Haematology, London, 13, 23

Hayashi N., Yoda B., Kikuchi G. (1969): Arch. Biochem. Biophys. 131, 83

Hayashi N., Yoda B., Kikuchi G. (1970): J. Biochem. 67, 859

Heilmeyer L., Keller W., Vivell O., Keiderling W., Betke K., Wöhler F., Schultze H. E. (1961): Dtsch. Med. Wschr. 96, 1745

Hemmaplardh D., Kailis S. G., Morgan E. H. (1974): Brit. J. Haemat. 28, 63

Hemmaplardh D., Morgan E. H. (1974): Biochim. biophys. Acta (Amst.) 373, 84

Hendrick D., Knöchel W., Schwarz W., Pitzel S., Tiedemann H. (1974a): Develop. Biol. 36, 299

184

Hendrick D., Schwarz W., Pizel S., Tiedemann H. (1974b): Biochim. biophys. Acta (Amst.) *340*, 278

Hershko C., Karsai A., Eylon L., Izak G. (1970): Blood *36*, 321

Heywood J. D. (1967): Clin. Res. *15*, 279

Heywood J. D., Finch C. A. (1970): Proc. Soc. exp. Biol. Med. *134*, 131

Heywood J. D., Karon M., Weissman S. (1965): J. Lab. clin. Med. *66*, 476

Heywood J. D., Karon M., Weissman S. (1966): J. Lab. clin. Med. *67*, 246

Heywood S. M. (1970a): Nature (Lond.) *225*, 696

Heywood S. M. (1970b): Proc. nat. Acad. Sci. (Wash.) *67*, 1782

Heywood S. M., Thompson W. C. (1971): Biochem. biophys. Res. Commun. *43*, 470

Hillmann R. S. (1969): Ann. N.Y. Acad. Sci. *165*, (Art 1), 100

Hillman R. S. (1970): Factors affecting hemoglobin regeneration. In: Iron Deficiency. (Eds. Hallberg L., Harwerth H.-G. and Vannotti A.), Academic Press, London and New York, p. 531

Hines J. D. (1969): J. Lab. clin. Med. *74*, 882

Hines J. D., Grasso J. A. (1970): Seminars Haemat. *7*, 86

Hoerz W., McCarty K. S. (1969): Proc. nat. Acad. Sci. (Wash.) *63*, 1206

Holder J. W., Lingrel J. B. (1970): Biochim. biophys. Acta (Amst.) *204*, 210

Holtz P., Palm D. (1964): Pharmacol. Rev. *16*, 113

Honig G. R. (1967): J. clin. Invest. *46*, 1778

Honig G. R., Rowan B. Q., Mason R. G. (1969): J. biol. Chem. *244*, 2027

Hori M., Fisher J. M., Rabinovitz M. (1967): Science *155*, 83

Hori M., Rabinovitz M. (1968): Proc. nat. Acad. Sci. (Wash.) *59*, 1349

Hosain F., Finch C. A. (1964): J. Lab. clin. Med. *64*, 905

Housman D., Forget B. G., Skoultchi A., Benz E. J. Jr. (1973): Proc. nat. Acad. Sci. (Wash.) *70*, 1809

Housman D., Jacobs-Lorena M., Rajbhandary U. L., Lodish H. F. (1970): Nature (Lond.) *227*, 913

Housman D., Pemberton R., Taber R. (1971): Proc. nat. Acad. Sci. (Wash.) *68*, 2716

Howard G. A., Adamson S. D., Herbert E. (1970a): J. biol. Chem. *245*, 6237

Howard G. A., Adamson S. D., Herbert E. (1970b): Biochim. biophys. Acta (Amst.) *213*, 237

Howard G. A., Traugh J. A., Croser E. A., Traut R. R. (1975): J. mol. Biol. *93*, 391

Hrinda M. E., Goldwasser E. (1969): Biochim. biophys. Acta (Amst.) *195*, 165

Huehns E. R., Shooter E. M. (1965): J. Med. Gen. *2*, 48

Huez G., Burny A., Marbaix G., Schram E. (1967): Europ. J. Biochem. *1*, 179

Huez G., Marbaix G., Hubert E., Cleuter Y., Leclercq M., Chantrenne H., Devos R., Soreq H., Nudel U., Littauer U. Z. (1975): Europ. J. Biochem. *59*, 589

Huez G., Marbaix G., Hubert E., Leclerq M., Nudel U., Soreq H., Salomon R., Lebleu B., Revel M., Littauer U. Z. (1974): Proc. nat. Acad. Sci (Wash.) *71*, 3143

Huez G., Marbaix G., Nokin P., Cleuter Y. (1976): 8th International Berlin Symposium on Structure and Function of Erythrocytes. Abstracts, p. 27

Humphries S. (1974): Biochem. biophys. Res. Commun. *58*, 927

Hunt J. A. (1970): Nature (Lond.) *226*, 950

Hunt T., Hunter T., Munro A. (1968a): J. mol. Biol. *36*, 31

Hunt R. T., Hunter A. R., Munro A. J. (1968b): Nature (Lond.) *220*, 481

Hunt T., Hunter T., Munro A. (1969a): J. mol. Biol. *43*, 123

Hunt R. T., Hunter A. R., Munro A. J. (1969b): Proc. Nutr. Soc. *28*, 248

Hunt T., Vanderhoff G., London I. M. (1972): J. mol. Biol. *66*, 471

Hunter A. R., Jackson R. J. (1975): Europ. J. Biochem. *58*, 421

Imaizumi T., Diggelmann H., Scherrer K. (1973): Proc. nat. Acad. Sci. (Wash.) *70*, 1122

Ingram V. M. (1963): The Hemoglobins in Genetics and Evolution. Columbia University Press, New York

Inouye A., Shinagawa Y., Masumura S. (1963): Nature (Lond.) *199*, 1290

Irving E. A., Elliott W. H. (1969): Proc. Austral. Biochem. Soc., 13th Ann. Meeting, p. 170

Iscove N. N. (1975) In: Erythropoiesis. Proceedings of the Fourth International Conference on Erythropoiesis (Ed. by Nakao K., Fisher J. W. and Takaku F.), University of Tokyo Press, p. 165

Iscove N. N., Sieber F. (1975): Exp. Hemat. *3*, 32

Israels L. G., Yoda B., Schacter B. A. (1975): Ann. N.Y. Acad. Sci. *244*, 651

Itano H. A. (1965) In: Abnormal haemoglobins in Africa. CIOMS Symposium. (Ed. by J. H. P. Jonxis). Blackwell Scient. Publ. Ltd., Oxford, p. 3

Iyer G. Y. N. (1968): Brit. J. Haemat. *15*, 561

Jackson R., Hunter T. (1970): Nature (Lond.) *227*, 672

Jacob F., Monod J. (1961): J. mol. Biol. *3*, 318

Jacobs A. (1974) In: Iron in Biochemistry and Medicine (Ed. by Jacobs A. and Worwood M.) Academic Press, London and New York

Jacobs A., Miller F., Worwood M., Beamish M. R., Wardrop C. A. J. (1972): Brit. Med. J. *4*, 206

Jacobs-Lorena M., Baglioni C. (1972): Proc. nat. Acad. Sci. (Wash.) *69*, 1425

Jandl J. H., Inman J. K., Simmons R. L., Allen D. W. (1959): J. clin. Invest. *38*, 161

Jandl J. H., Katz J. H. (1963): J. clin. Invest. *42*, 314

Jensen W. W., Moreno G. (1964): C.R. Acad. Sci. (Paris) *258*, 3596

Jones M. S., Jones O. T. G. (1969): Biochem. J. *113*, 507

Jones M. S., Jones O. T. G. (1970): Biochem. biophys. Res. Commun, *41*, 1072

Jones O. P. (1964): Anat. Rec. *148*, 296

Jones O. P. (1965): J. nat. Cancer Inst. *35*, 139

Kabat D. (1970): Biochemistry *9*, 4160

Kabat D. (1971): Biochemistry *10*, 197

Kabat D. (1975): J. biol. Chem. *250*, 6085

Kacian D. L., Spiegelman S., Bank A., Terada M., Metafora S., Dow L., Marks P. A. (1972): Nature New Biol. *235*, 167

Kacian D. L., Gambino R., Dow L. W., Grossbard E., Natta E., Ramirez E., Spiegelman S., Marks P. A., Bank A. (1973): Proc. nat. Acad. Sci. (Wash.) *70*, 1886

Kadenbach B. (1970): Europ. J. Biochem. *12*, 392

Kaempfer R., Kaufman J. (1972): Proc. nat. Acad. Sci. (Wash.) *69*, 3317

Kailis S. G., Morgan E. H. (1974): Brit. J. Haemat. *28*, 37

Kappas A., Bradlow H. L., Gilette P. N., Gallagher T. F. (1972): J. exp. Med. *136*, 1043

Kappas A., Levere R. D., Granick S. (1968): Semin. Hematol. *5*, 323

Kappas A., Song Ch. S., Levere R. D., Sachson R. A., Granick S. (1968): Proc. nat. Acad. Sci. (Wash.) *61/2*, 509

Karibian D., London I. M. (1965): Bioch. biophys. Res. Commun. *18*, 243

Kark J. A., Haut M. S., Duffy T. P., McQuilkin C. T., Hicks C. U. (1975): Abstr. International Soc. of Haematology, London, *13*, 11

Katz J. H. (1965): Series Haematol. *6*, 15

Katz J. H. (1970) In: Regulation of Hematopoiesis (Ed. by A. S. Gordon), Vol. 1, Allpeton-Century-Crofts, New York, p. 539

Katz J. H., Jandl J. H. (1964) In: Iron Metabolism (Ed. by F. Gross). Springer Verlag, Berlin, p. 103

Kazazian H. H. Jr., Freedman M. L. (1968): J. biol. Chem. *243*, 6446

Kazazian H. H., Snyder P. G., Cheng T. (1974): Biochim. biophys. Res. Commun. *59*, 1053

Kikuchi G., Ja Kim H., Watari K., Tomita Y., Ohashi A. (1973): Enzyme *16*, 258

Kikuchi G., Kuman A., Talmage P., Shemin D. (1958): J. biol. Chem. *233*, 1274

Kikuchi G., Yoshida T. (1975) In: International Conference on Porphyrin Metabolism, Samxäs, Finland, p. 14

King H. W. S., Gould H. J., Shearman J. J. (1971): J. mol. Biol. 61, 143

Klein J. R. (1961): Amer. J. Physiol. *201*, 663

Klein J. R. (1968): Arch. Biochem. Biophys. *127*, 666

Knöchel W., Hendrick D., Schröter S., Tiedermann H. (1973): Hoppe-Seyler's Z. physiol. Chem. *354*, 1389

Koller M. E., Prante P. H., Ulvik R., Romslo I. (1976): Biochem. biophys. Res. Commun. 71, 339

Komatsu U., Feeney R. E. (1967): Biochemistry 6, 1136

Konopka K., Leyko W., Gondko R., Sidorczyk Z., Fabjanowska Z., Swedowska M. (1969): Clin. chim. Acta *359*, 66

Konopka K., Szotor M. (1972): Acta haemat. *47*, 157

Kornfeld S. (1968) In: XII Congress International Society of Hematology, New York

Kornfeld S. (1969): Biochim. biophys. Acta (Amst.) 194, 25

Kosower N. S., Vanderhoff G. A., Benerofe B., Hunt T., Kosower E. M. (1971): Biochem. biophys. Res. Commun. *45*, 816

Kosower N. S., Vanderhoff G. A., Kosower E. M. (1972): Biochim. biophys. Acta (Amst.) *272*, 623

Krantz S. B. (1973): J. Lab. clin. Med. *82*, 847

Krantz S. B., Goldwasser E. (1965): Biochim. biophys. Acta (Amst.) *103*, 325

Krantz S. B., Jacobson L. O. (1970): Erythropoietin and the Regulation of Erythropoiesis. The University of Chicago Press, Chicago and London

Krueger R. C., Melnick I., Klein J. R. (1956): Arch. Biochem. Biophys. *64*, 302

Kruh J., Borsook H. (1956): J. biol. Chem. 220, 905

Kruh J., Dreyfus J. C., Schapira G. (1964): Biochim. biophys. Acta (Amst.) *87*, 253

Kuchinskas E. J., Horvath A., Du Vigneaud V. (1957): Arch. Biochem. Biophys. *68*, 69

Kurashima Y., Hayashi N., Kikuchi G. (1970): J. Biochem. (Tokyo) *67*, 863

Kushner J. P., Barbuto A. J. (1974): Clin. Res. *22*, 178

Labbe R. F. (1967): Lancet *i*, 1361

Labbe R. F., Nutter J., Cowger M. L. (1969): Biochem. Med. *3*, 210

Labbe R. F., Nutter J., Cowger M. L., Nielsen L. D. (1970): Biochem. Med. *3*, 465

Labbe R. F., Hubbard N. (1960): Biochim. biophys. Acta (Amst.) *41*, 185

Labrie F. (1969): Nature (Lond.) *221*, 1217

187

Ladhoff A.-M., Thiele B. J., Coutelle C. (1975): Europ. J. Biochem. *58*, 431

Lahey M. E., Gubler C. S., Chose M. S., Cartwright G. E., Wintrobe M. M. (1952): Blood 7, 1053

Lajtha L. G. (1957): Physiol. Rev. *37*, 52

Lajtha L. G. (1963): J. cell. comp. Physiol., Suppl. 1, *67*, 143

Lajtha L. G. (1975): Brit. J. Haemat. *29*, 529

Lajtha L. G., Suit H. D. (1955): Brit. J. Haemat. *1*, 55

Lamform H., Knopf P. M. (1964): J. mol. Biol. *9*, 558

Lane C. D., Gurdon J. B., Woodland H. R. (1974): Nature (Lond.) *25*, 436

Lane C. D., Marbaix G., Gurdon J. B. (1971): J. mol. Biol. *61*, 73

Lane R. S. (1971): Biochim. biophys. Acta (Amst.) *243*, 193

Lane R. S. (1972): Brit. J. Haemat. *22*, 309

Lane R. S., Finch C. A. (1970): Clin. Sci. *38*, 783

Lang A., Lehmann H., King-Lewis P. A. (1974): Nature (Lond.) *249*, 467

Langelaan D. E., Losowsky M. S., Toothill C. (1969): Clin. chim. Acta *26*, 245

Langelaan E. D., Losowsky M. S., Toothill C. (1970): Clin. chim. Acta *27*, 453

Langridge R. (1963): Science *140*, 1000

Lanyon W. G., Ottolenghi S., Williamson R. (1975): Proc. nat. Acad. Sci. (Wash.) *72*, 258

Lanyon W. G., Paul J., Williamson R. (1972): Europ. J. Biochem. *31*, 38

Lascelles J. (1957): Biochem. J. *66*, 65

Lascelles J. (1960): J. gen. Microbiol. *23*, 487

Lascelles J. (1968): The regulation of haem and chlorophyll synthesis. In: Porphyrins and Related Compounds. (Ed. Goodwin T. W.) Academic Press, London and New York, p. 49

Laußberger V. (1936): Čas. Lék. čes. *75*, 1535

Laußberger V. (1937): Bull. Soc. Chim. Biol. *19*, 1575

Laver W. G., Neuberger A., Udenfriend S. (1958): Biochem. J. 70, 4

Lebleu B., Marbaix G., Huez G., Temmermen J., Butny A., Chantrenne H. (1971): Europ. J. Biochem. *19*, 264

Lebleu B., Marbaix G., Werenne J., Burny A., Huez G. (1970): Biochem. biophys. Res. Commun. *40*, 731

Lebleu B., Nudel U., Falcoff E., Prives C., Revel M. (1972): FEBS Letters *25*, 97

Legon S., Brayley A., Hunt T., Jackson R. J. (1974): Biochem. biophys. Res. Commun. *56*, 745

Legon S., Jackson R. J., Hunt T. (1973): Nature New Biol. *241*, 150

Lehmann H., Huntsman R. G. (1974): Man's Haemoglobins, 2nd revised edition, North-Holland Publishing Co., Amsterdam and Oxford

Lehmann H., Lang A. (1974): Ann. N.Y. Acad. Sci. 232, 152

Levin D. H., Ranu R. S., Ernst V., Fifer M. A., London I. M. (1975): Proc. nat. Acad. Sci. (Wash.) *72*, 4849

Levin E. Y., Coleman D. L. (1967): J. biol. Chem. *242*, 4248

Lichtman H. C., Feldman F. (1967): Proc. Soc. exp. Biol. (N. Y.) *126*, 38

Lim L., Canellakis E. S. (1970): Nature (Lond.) *227*, 710

Lindberg U., Persson T. (1972): Europ. J. Biochem. *31*, 246

Lingrel J. B., Lockard R. E., Jones A. F., Burr H. E., Holder J. W. (1971): Ser. Haemat. *4*, 37

Lingrel J. B., Woodland H. R. (1974): Europ. J. Biochem. *47*, 47

Litt M., Kabat D. (1972): J. biol. Chem. *247*, 6659

188

Littlefield J. W., Keller E. B., Gross J., Zamecnik P. C. (1955): J. biol. Chem. *217*, 111
Lochhead A. C., Kramer G., Goldberg A. (1963): Brit. J. Haemat. *9*, 39
Lockard R. E., Lingrel J. B. (1969): Biochem. biophys. Res. Commun. *37*, 204
Lockard R. E., Lingrel J. B. (1971): Nature New Biol. *233*, 204
Lodish H. F. (1971): J. biol. Chem. *246*, 7131
Lodish H. F. (1973): Proc. nat. Acad. Sci. (Wash.) *70*, 1526
Lodish H. F., Desalu O. (1973): J. biol. Chem. *248*, 3520
Lodish H. F., Jacobsen M. (1972): J. biol. Chem. *247*, 3622
Lodish H. F., Nathan D. G. (1972): J. biol. Chem. *247*, 7822
London I. M., Bruns G. P., Karibian D. (1964): Medicine *43*, 789
London I. M., Shemin D., Rittenberg D. (1950): J. biol. Chem. *183*, 749
Lorkin P. A., Lang A. (1976): Brit. med. Bull. *32*, 239
Lubsen N. H., Davis B. D. (1972): Proc. nat. Acad. Sci. (Wash.) *69*, 353
Lubsen N. H., Davis B. D. (1974): Biochim. biophys. Acta (Amst.) *335*, 196
Lucas-Lenard J., Lipmann F. (1971): Ann. Rev. Biochem. *40*, 409
Lukanidin E. M., Georgiev G. P., Williamson R. (1971): FEBS Letters *19*, 152
Lumeng L., Li T. K. (1974): J. clin. Invest. *53*, 693
Luppis B., Bargellesi A., Conconi F. (1970): Biochemistry *21*, 4175
Malinowska T., Mazanowska A., Dancewicz A. M., Kowalski E. (1964): Bull. Acad. pol. Sci. *12*, 59
Maines M. D., Kappas A. (1976): Biochem. J. *154*, 125
Maniatias G. M., Rifkind R. A., Bank A., Marks P. A. (1973): Proc. nat. Acad. Sci. (Wash.) *70*, 3189
Mansbridge J. N., Crossley J. A., Lanyon W. G., Williamson R. (1974): Europ. J. Biochem. *44*, 261
Manyan D. R., Arimura G. K., Yunis A. A. (1972): J. Lab. clin. Med. *79*, 137
Manyan D. R., Yunis A. A. (1970): Biochem. biophys. Res. Commun. *41*, 926
Marbaix G., Burny A. (1964): Biochem. biophys. Res. Commun. *16*, 522
Marbaix G., Burny A., Huez G., Chantrenne H. (1966): Biochim. biophys. Acta (Amst.) *114*, 404
Marbaix G., Gurdon J. B. (1972): Biochim. biophys. Acta (Amst.) *281*, 86
Marbaix G., Huez G., Burny A., Cleuter Y., Hubert E., Leclercq M., Chantrenne H., Soreq H., Nudel U., Littauer U. Z. (1975): Proc. nat. Acad. Sci. (Wash.) *72*, 3065
Marbaix G., Huez G., Burny A., Hubert E., Leclercq M., Cleuter Y., Chantrenne H., Soreq H., Nudel U., Littauer U. (1976): 8th International Berlin Symposium on Structure and Function of Erythrocytes. Abstracts, p. 6
Marbaix G., Lane C. D. (1972): J. mol. Biol. *67*, 517
Marks P. A., Burka E. R., Schlessinger D. (1962): Proc. nat. Acad. Sci. (Wash.) *48*, 2163
Marotta C. A., Forget B. G., Weissman S. M., Verma I. M., McCaffrey R. P., Baltimore D. (1974): Proc. nat. Acad. Sci. (Wash.) *71*, 2300
Martinez-Medellin J. (1972): Ph. D. Dissertation. University of California, San Diego, Calif.
Martinez-Medellin J., Schulman H. M. (1972): Biochim. biophys. Acta (Amst.) *264*, 272
Martinez-Medellin J., Schulman H. M. (1973): Biochim. biophys. Res. Commun. *53*, 32
Martini O. H. W., Gould H. J. (1973): Biochim. biophys. Acta (Amst.) *295*, 621
Marver H. S., Collins A., Tschudy D. P., Rechcigl M. Jr. (1966): J. biol. Chem. *241*, 4323
Marver H. S., Schmid R., Schützel H. (1968): Biochem. biophys. Res. Commun. *33*, 969

Marver H. S., Tschudy D. P., Perlroth M. G., Collins A. (1966): J. biol. Chem. *241*, 2803

Mathews M. B. (1972): Biochim. biophys. Acta (Amst.) *272*, 168

Mathews M. B., Hunt T., Brayley A. (1973): Nature New Biol. *243*, 230

Mathews M. B., Korner A. (1970): Europ. J. Biochem. *17*, 328

Mathews M. B., Osborn M., Lingrel J. B. (1971): Nature New Biol. *233*, 206

Mathews M. B., Pragnell I. B., Osborn M., Arnstein H. R. V. (1972): Biochim. biophys. Acta (Amst.) *287*, 113

Mathias A. P., Williamson R. (1964): J. mol. Biol. *9*, 498

Mathias A. P., Williamson R., Huxley H. E., Prage S. (1964): J. mol. Biol. *9*, 154

Matioli G. T., Eylar E. M. (1964): Proc. nat. Acad. Sci. (Wash.) *52*, 508

Mauzerall D. (1964): J. Pediat. *64*, 5

Maxwell C. R., Kamper C. S., Rabinovitz M. (1971): J. mol. Biol. *58*, 317

Maxwell C. R., Rabinovitz M. (1969): Biochem. biophys. Res. Commun. *35*, 79

Mazanowska A., Pancewicz A. M., Malinowska T., Kowalski E. (1969): Europ. J. Biochem. *7*, 583

Mazanowska A. M., Neuberger A., Tait G. H. (1966): Biochem. J. *98*, 117

Mazur A., Carleton, Anne (1963): J. biol. Chem. *238*, 1817

Mazur A., Green S., Carleton A. (1960): J. biol. Chem. *235/3*, 595

McKay R., Druyan R., Getz G. S., Rabinovitz M. (1969): Biochem. J. *114*, 455

McKeehan W. D. (1974): J. biol. Chem. *249*, 6517

McKeehan W. L., Hardesty B. (1969): J. biol. Chem. *244*, 4330

Merrick W. C., Graf H., Anderson W. F. (1974) In: Methods in Enzymology (Ed. by Moldave K. and Grossman L.) Vol. 30 (P.F.) Academic Press, New York and London, p. 128

Merrick W. C., Kemper W. M., Anderson W. F. (1975): J. biol. Chem. *250*, 5556

Merrick W. C., Lubsen N. H., Anderson W. F. (1973): Proc. nat. Acad. Sci. (Wash.) *70*, 2220

Metafora S., Terada M., Dow L. W., Marks P. A., Bank A. (1972): Proc. nat. Acad. Sci. (Wash.) *69*, 1299

Meyer U. A., Marver H. S. (1971): Science *171*, 64

Miller R. L., Schweet R. (1968): Arch. Biochem. Biophys. *125*, 632

Milner P. F., Clegg J. B., Weatherall D. J. (1971): Lancet *1*, 729

Mirand E. A. (1965): Nat. Cancer Inst. Monograph *22*, 483

Mirand E. A. (1967): Proc. Soc. exp. Biol. (N.Y.) *125*, 562

Mirand E. A., Steeves R. A., McGarry M. P. (1971) In: The Regulation of Erythropoiesis and Haemoglobin Synthesis. (Ed. by Trávníček T. and Neuwirt J.) Universita Karlova, Praha, p. 165

Mitchell B. S., Adamson J. W. (1975) In: Erythropoiesis. Proceedings of the Fourth International Conference on Erythropoiesis (Ed. by Nakao K., Fisger J. W. and Takaku, F.), University of Tokyo Press, p. 151

Mizuno S., Fisher J. M., Rabinovitz M. (1972): Biochim. biophys. Acta (Amst.) *272*, 638

Mizuno S., Rabinovitz M. (1973): Proc. nat. Acad. Sci. (Wash.) *70*, 787

Moar V. A., Gurdon J. B., Lane C. D., Marbaix G. (1971): J. mol. Biol. *61*, 93

Mollin D. L., MacGibbon B. H. (1972): Brit. J. Haemat. *23* (Suppl.) 147

Moores R. R., Stohlman F. Jr., Brecher G. (1963): Blood *22*, 286

Morel C., Kayibanda B., Scherrer K. (1971): FEBS Letters *18*, 84

Morgan E. H. (1964): Brit. J. Haemat. *10/4*, 442

Morgan E. H. (1971): Biochim. biophys. Acta (Amst.) *244*, 103

Morgan E. H. (1974) In: Iron in Biochemistry and Medicine (Ed. by Jacobs A. and Worwood M.), Academic Press, London and New York, p. 29

Morgan E. H., Appleton T. C. (1969): Nature (Lond.) *223*, 1371

Morgan E. H., Baker E. (1969): Biochim. biophys. Acta (Amst.) *184*, 442

Morgan E. H., Baker E. (1974): Biochim. biophys. Acta (Amst.) *363*, 240

Morgan E. H., Laurell, C.-B. (1963): Brit. J. Haemat. *9*, 171

Morris A. J., Liang K. (1968): Arch. Biochem. Biophys. *125*, 468

Morrison M., Brinkley S., Gorski J., Lingrel J. B. (1974): J. biol. Chem. *249*, 5290

Morrison M. R., Gorski J., Lingrel J. B. (1972): Biochem. biophys. Res. Commun. *49*, 775

Mushinski J. F., Galizzi A., Von Ehrenstein G. (1970): Biochemistry *9*, 489

Myhre E. (1964a): Scand. J. clin. Lab. Invest. *16*, 201

Myhre E. (1964b): Scand. J. clin. Lab. Invest. *16*, 212

Najean Y. (1961): Path. et Biol. *9*, 1573

Najean Y., Ardaillou N., Bernard J. (1960): Rev. franc. Etudes clin. et biol. *5*, 783

Najean Y., Ardaillou N., Mulmann M. (1964): Nouv. Rev. franc. Hématol. *4*, 31

Najean Y., Dresch C., Ardaillou N., Bernard J. (1967): Amer. J. Physiol. *213*, 533

Nakao K., Sassa S., Wasa O., Takaku F. (1968): Ann. N.Y. Acad. Sci. *149*, 224

Näslund P. H., Hultin T. (1970): Biochim. biophys. Acta (Amst.) *204*, 237

Näslund P. H., Hultin T. (1971): Biochim. biophys. Acta (Amst.) *254*, 104

Nathan D. G., Lodish H. F., Kan Y. W., Housman D. (1971): Proc. nat. Acad. Sci. (Wash.) *68*, 2514

Naughton N. A., Dintzis H. M. (1962): Proc. nat. Acad. Sci. (Wash.) *48*, 1822

Necheles T. F. (1971) In: The Regulation of Erythropoiesis and Haemoglobin Synthesis. (Ed. by Trávníček T. and Neuwirt J.) Universita Karlova, Praha, p. 292

Neuberger A. (1961): Biochem. J. *78*, 1

Neuberger A., Sandy J. D., Tait G. H. (1973): Enzyme *16*, 79

Neuwirt J., Borová J., Poňka P. (1968): FEBS Letters *1*, 209

Neuwirt J., Borová J., Poňka P. (1975a) In: Proteins of Iron Storage and Transport in Biochemistry and Medicine (Ed. by Crichton R. R.) North-Holland Publishing Company, Amsterdam, p. 161

Neuwirt J., Poňka P. (1972) In: Synthesis, Structure and Function of Hemoglobin (Ed. by Martin H. and Nowicki L.), J. F. Lehmanns Verlag, München, p. 61

Neuwirt J., Poňka P., Borová J. (1969a): Europ. J. Biochem. *9*, 36

Neuwirt J., Poňka P., Borová J. (1971) In: The Regulation of Erythropoiesis and Haemoglobin Synthesis (Ed. by Trávníček T. and Neuwirt J.) Universita Karlova, Praha, p. 357

Neuwirt J., Poňka P., Borová J. (1972): Biochim. biophys. Acta (Amst.) *264*, 235

Neuwirt J., Poňka P., Borová J. (1975b) In: Erythropoiesis. Proceedings of the Fourth International Conference on Erythropoiesis (Ed. by Nakao, K., Fisher J. W. and Takaku F.), University of Tokyo Press, p. 413

Neuwirt J., Poňka P., Borová J., Prchal J. F. (1969b): Blut *19*, 17

Nicol A. G., Conkie D., Lanyon W. G., Drewienkiewicz C. E., Williamson R., Paul J.: Biochim. biophys. Acta (Amst.) *277*, 342

Nienhuis A. W., Anderson W. F. (1971): J. clin. Invest. *50*, 2458

Nienhuis A. W., Anderson W. F. (1972): Proc. nat. Acad. Sci. (Wash.) *69*, 2184

Nienhuis A. W., Canfield P. H., Anderson W. F. (1973): J. clin. Invest. *52*, 1735

Nienhuis A. W., Falvey A. K., Anderson W. F. (1974) In: Methods in Enzymology (Ed. by Moldave K. and Grossman L.) Vol. 30 (P.F.), Academic Press, New York and London, p. 621

Nirenberg M., Leder P., Berryfield M., Brimacombe R., Trupin J., Rottman F., O'Neal C. (1965): Proc. nat. Acad. Sci. (Wash.) *53*, 1161

Nokin P., Burny A., Cleuter Y., Huez G., Marbaix G., Chantrenne H. (1975): Europ. J. Biochem. *53*, 83

Nokin P., Gautier F. (1973): Mol. Biol. Rep. *1*, 47

Nokin P., Huez G., Marbaix G., Burny A., Chantrenne H. (1976): Europ. J. Biochem. *62*, 509

Noyes W. D., Hosain F., Finch C. A. (1964): J. Lab. clin. Med. *64*, 574

Nudel U., Lebleu B., Revel M. (1973): Proc. nat. Acad. Sci. (Wash.) *70*, 2139

Nudel U., Soreq H., Littauer U. Z., Marbaix G., Huez G., Leclercq M., Hubert E., Chantrenne H. (1976): Europ. J. Biochem. *64*, 115

Olsen G. D., Gaskill P., Kabat D. (1972): Biochim. biophys. Acta (Amst.) *272*, 297

Osaki S., Johnson D. A., Frieden E. (1966): J. biol. Chem. *241*, 2746

Ottolenghi S., Lanyon W. G., Paul J., Williamson R., Weatherall D. J., Clegg J. B., Pritchard J., Pootrakul J., Wong Hock Boon (1974): Nature (Lond.) *251*, 389

Packman S., Aviv H., Ross J., Leder P. (1972): Biochem. biophys. Res. Commun. *49*, 813

Paul J., Hunter J. A. (1969): J. mol. Biol. *42*, 31

Pemberton R. E., Baglioni C. (1973): J. mol. Biol. *81*, 255

Pemberton R. E., Housman D., Lodish H. F., Baglioni C. (1972): Nature New Biol. *235*, 99

Perlroth M. G., Tschudy D. P., Marver H. S., Beard C. W., Zeigel R. F., Rechzigl M., Collins A. (1966): Amer. J. Med. *41*, 149

Perry R. P., Scherrer K. (1975): FEBS Letters *57*, 73

Pestka S. (1971): Ann. Rev. Biochem. *40*, 697

Piantadosi C. A., Dickerman H. W., Spivak J. L. (1976): J. clin. Invest. *57*, 20

Picciano D. J., Prichard P. M., Merrick W. C., Shafritz D. A., Graf H., Crystal R. G., Anderson W. F. (1973): J. biol. Chem. *248*, 204

Pinelli A., Capuano A. (1973): Enzyme *16*, 203

Pollycove M. (1964) In: Iron Metabolism (Ed. by F. Gross) Berlin, Springer Verlag, p. 148

Pollycove M., Mortimer R. (1961): J. clin. Invest. *40*, 753

Poňka P., Borová J., Neuwirt J. (1973b): Biochim. biophys. Acta (Amst.) *304*, 715

Poňka, P., Fuchs O., Borová J., Neuwirt J., Nečas E. (1977a): Acta Biol. Med. Germ. (in press)

Poňka P., Neuwirt J. (1969): Blood *33*, 690

Poňka P., Neuwirt J. (1970): Brit. J. Haemat. *19/5*, 593

Poňka P., Neuwirt J. (1971): Biochim. biophys. Acta (Amst.) *230/2*, 381

Poňka P., Neuwirt J. (1971b) In: The Regulation of Erythropoiesis and Haemoglobin Synthesis (Ed. by Trávníček T. and Neuwirt J.), Universita Karlova, Praha, p. 326

Poňka P., Neuwirt J. (1972): Experientia *28/2*, 189

Poňka P., Neuwirt J. (1974): Brit. J. Haemat. *28*, 1

Poňka P., Neuwirt J. (1975a) In: Proteins of Iron Storage and Transport in Biochemistry and Medicine (Ed. by Crichton R. R.). North-Holland Publishing Company, Amsterdam, p. 147

Poňka P., Neuwirt J. (1975b): New Engl. J. Med. *293*, 406

Poňka P., Neuwirt J., Borová J. (1973): Biochim. biophys. Acta (Amst.) *304*, 123

Poňka P., Neuwirt J., Borová J. (1974): Enzyme *17*, 91

Poňka P., Neuwirt J., Borová J. (1975) In: Erythropoiesis. Proceedings of the Fourth International Conference on Erythropoiesis (Ed. by Nakao K., Fisher J. W. and Takaku F.) University of Tokyo Press, p. 403

Poňka P., Neuwirt J., Borová J., Fuchs O. (1977b) In: Iron Metabolism. Ciba Foundation Symposium 51 (new series). Elsevier-Excerpta Medica-North Holland, Amsterdam (in press)

Poňka P., Neuwirt J., Sperl M., Březík Z. (1970): Biochem. biophys. Res. Commun. *38*, 817

Porra R. J., Barnes R., Jones O. T. G. (1973): Enzyme *16*, 1

Porra R. J., Jones O. T. G. (1963): Biochem. J. *87*, 186

Porra R. J., Ross B. D. (1965): Biochem. J. *94*, 557

Pragnell I. B., Arnstein H. R. V. (1970): FEBS Letters *9*, 331

Prather N., Ravel J. M., Hardesty B., Shive W. (1974): Biochem. biophys. Res. Commun. *57*, 578

Prato V., Mazza U., Bianco G., Battistini V. (1968a): Blut *17*, 14

Prchal J., Neuwirt J. (1968): Folia haemat. *90*, 120

Prichard P. M., Anderson W. F. (1974) In: Methods in Enzymology (Ed. by Moldave K. and Grossman L.), Vol. 30 (P.F.), Academic Press, New York and London, p. 136

Prichard P. M., Gilbert J. M., Shafritz D. A., Anderson W. F. (1970): Nature (Lond.) 226, 511

Prichard P. M., Picciano D. J., Laycock D. G., Anderson W. F. (1971): Proc. nat. Acad. Sci. (Wash.) *68*, 2752

Primosigh J. V., Thomas E. D. (1968): J. clin. Invest. *47*, 1473

Princiotto J. V., Rubin M., Shashaty G. C., Zapolski E. J. (1964): J. clin. Invest. *43*, 825

Protzel A., Morris A. J. (1973): J. biol. Chem. 248, 7438

Proudfoot N. J., Brownlee G. G. (1974): FEBS Letters *38*, 179

Rabinovitz M., Freedman M. L., Fischer J. M., Maxwell C. R. (1969): Cold Spring Harb. Symp. quant. Biol. *34*, 567

Rabinovitz M., Olson E. (1956): Exper. Cell Res. *10*, 747

Rabinovitz M., Waxman H. S. (1965): Nature (Lond.) *206*, 897

Rahamimoff H., Arnstein H. R. V. (1969): Biochem. J. *115*, 113

Ramirez F., Gambino R., Maniatis G. M., Rifkind R. A., Marks P. A., Bank A. (1975): J. biol. Chem. *250*, 6054

Reissmann K. R., Udupa K. B. (1972): Cell Tissue Kinet. *5*, 481

Rich A., Eikenberry E. F., Malkin L. I. (1966): Cold Spring Harb. Symp. quant. Biol. *31*, 303

Rieder R. F. (1972): J. clin. Invest. *51*, 364

Rieder R. F., Weatherall D. J. (1965): J. clin. Invest. *44*, 42

Riethmüller G., Tuppy H. (1964): Biochem. Ztschr. *340*, 413

Rifkind R. A., Bank A., Marks P. A. (1974) In: The Red Blood Cell, Second Edition (Ed. by Surgenor, D. M.) Vol. I, Academic Press, New York and London, p. 51

Riggs T. R., Walker R. M. (1963): J. biol. Chem. *238*, 2663

Rimington C. (1966): Acta med. Scand. *179*, Suppl. 445, 11

Rimington C., Booij H. L. (1957): Biochem. J. *65*, 3P

Ring K., Gross W., Heinz E. (1970): Arch. Biochem. Biophys. *137*, 243

Roberts B. E., Paterson B. M. (1973): Proc. nat. Acad. Sci. (Wash.) *70*, 2330

Roberts A. V., Weatherall D. J., Clegg J. B. (1972): Biochem. biophys. Res. Commun. *47*, 81

Romslo I. (1974): Biochim. biophys. Acta (Amst.) *357*, 34

Rosenberg A., Marcus O. (1974): Brit. J. Haemat. *26*, 79

Ross J., Aviv H., Scolnick E., Leder P. (1972a): Proc. nat. Acad. Sci. (Wash.) *69*, 264

Ross J., Ikawa Y., Leder P. (1972b): Proc. nat. Acad. Sci. (Wash.) *69*, 3620

Ross J., Sautner D. (1976): Cell 8, 520

Rychlík I., Šorm F. (1962): Collection Czechoslov. Chem. Commun. *27*, 2433

Safer B., Anderson W. F., Merrick W. C. (1975): J. biol. Chem. *250*, 9067

Salera V., Magnanelli P., d'Avino R., Zecca I., Matcovich, A. L. (1961): Proc. 8th Congress Europ. Soc. Haemat. Vienna, 240a

Sampson J., Borghetti A. F. (1972b): Nature New Biol. *238*, 200

Sampson J., Mathews M. B., Osborn M., Borghetti A. F. (1972a): Biochemistry *11*, 3636

Sano S., Inoue S., Tanabe Y., Sumiya C., Kioke S. (1959): Science *129*, 275

Sassa S. (1976): J. exp. Med. *143*, 305

Sassa S., Granick S. (1970): Proc. nat. Acad. Sci. (Wash.) *67*, 517

Sassa S., Granick S. (1971) In: The Regulation of Erythropoiesis and Haemoglobin Synthesis (Ed. by Trávníček T., and Neuwirt J.) Universita Karlova, Praha, p. 299

Sassa S., Granick S., Chang C., Kappas A. (1975) In: Erythropoiesis. Proceedings of the Fourth International Conference on Erythropoiesis (Ed. by Nakao K., Fisher J. W., and Takaku F.) University of Tokyo Press, p. 383

Schade A. L. (1961): Behringwerk-Mitteilungen *39*, 130

Schaeffer J., Favelukes G., Schweet R. (1964): Biochim. biophys. Acta (Amst.) *80*, 247

Schapira G., Dreyfus J. C., Maleknia N. (1968a): Biochem. biophys. Res. Commun. *32*, 558

Schapira G., Rosa J., Maleknia N., Padieu P. (1968b) In: Methods in Enzymology (Ed. by Grossman L. and Moldave, K.) Vol. 12 (P.B.), Academic Press, New York, p. 747

Schapira G., Vaquero C., Reibel L. (1973): Biochimie *55*, 183

Scher W., Holland J. G., Friend C. (1971): Blood *37*, 428

Scherrer K. (1967): Exp. biol. Med. *1*, 244

Scherrer K. (1973): Acta endocrin. *74* (Suppl. 180), 95

Scherrer K., Marcaud L. (1968): J. cell. Physiol. *72* (Suppl.), 181

Schmid R., McDonagh A. F. (1975): International Conference on Porphyrin Metabolism, Sannäs, Finland, p. 32

Scholnick P. L., Hammaker L. E., Marver H. S. (1969): Proc. nat. Acad. Sci. (Wash.) *63*, 65

Scholnick P., Marver H. S., Schmid R. (1971): J. clin. Invest. *50*, 203

Schreier M. H., Staehelin T. (1973a): Europ. J. Biochem. *34*, 213

Schreier M. H., Staehelin T. (1973b): Proc. nat. Acad. Sci. (Wash.) *70*, 462

Schreier M. H., Staehelin T. (1973c): J. mol. Biol. *73*, 329

Schreier M. H., Staehelin T. (1973d): Nature New Biol. *242*, 35

Schreml W., Burka E. R. (1968): J. biol. Chem. *243*, 3573

Schroeder W. A., Huisman T. H. J., Shelton R., Shelton J. B., Kleihauer E. F., Dozy A. M., Robberson B. (1968): Proc. nat. Acad. Sci. (Wash.) *60*, 537

Schulman H. M. (1968): Biochim. biophys. Acta (Amst.) *155*, 253

Schulman H. M. (1975): Biochim. biophys. Acta (Amst.) *414*, 161

Schulman H. M., Martinez-Medellin J., Sidloi R. (1974): Biochim. biophys. Acta (Amst.) *343*, 529

194

Schulman H. M., Martinez-Medellin J., Sidloi R. (1974b): Biochim. biophys. Res. Commun. *56*, 220

Schulman M. P., Richert D. A. (1957): J. biol. Chem. *226*, 181

Schwartz H. C., Cartwright G. E., Smith E. L., Wintrobe M. M. (1959): Blood *14*, 486

Schweet R., Lamform H., Allen E. (1958): Proc. nat. Acad. Sci. (Wash.) *44*, 1029

Schweiger H. A. (1962): Int. Rev. Cytol. *13*, 135

Seid-Akhavan M., Winter W. P., Abramson R. K., Rucknagel D. L. (1972): Blood *40*, 927

Seip M., Gjessing L. R., Lie S. O. (1971): Scand. J. Haemat. *8*, 505

Seno S. (1966): Acta pathol. Japon. *16*, 457

Shaeffer J. R. (1967): Biochem. biophys. Res. Commun. *28*, 647

Shaeffer J. R., Trostle P. K., Evans R. F. (1967): Science *158*, 488

Shaeffer J. R., Trostle P. K., Evans R. F. (1969): J. biol. Chem. *244*, 4284

Shafritz D. A., Anderson W. F. (1970): J. biol. Chem. *245*, 5553

Shafritz D. A., Prichard P. M., Gilbert J. M., Anderson W. F. (1970): Biochem. biophys. Res. Commun. *38*, 721

Shafritz D. A., Prichard P. M., Gilbert J. M., Merrick W. C., Anderson W. F. (1972): Proc. nat. Acad. Sci. (Wash.) *69*, 983

Sheldon R., Jurale C., Kates J. (1972): Proc. nat. Acad. Sci. (Wash.) *69*, 417

Shemin D. (1970): Naturwissenschaften *57*, 185

Shemin D., Kumin S. (1952): J. biol. Chem. *198*, 827

Shemin D., London I. M., Rittenberg D. (1948): J. biol. Chem. *173*, 799

Shemin D., Rittenberg D. (1946): J. biol. Chem. *166*, 621

Shemin D., Russell Ch. (1954): J. Amer. chem. Soc. *76*, 1204

Sherman J. J., Hamlyn P. H., Gould H. J. (1974): FEBS Letters *47*, 171

Silverstein E. (1962): Biochem. Pharmacol. *11*, 431

Skoultchi A. I. (1975): Progr. clin. biol. Res. *1* (Erythrocyte Struc. Funct.), 121

Slabaugh R. C., Morris A. J. (1970): J. biol. Chem. *245*, 6182

Sly D. A., Grohlich D., Berkorovainy A. (1975a): Biochim. biophys. Acta (Amst.) *385*, 36

Sly D. A., Grohlich D., Berkorovainy A. (1975b) In: Proteins of Iron Storage and Medicine (Ed. by Crichton R. R.) North-Holland Publishing Company, Amsterdam, p. 141

Smith D. W. E. (1971): Science *171*, 577

Smith D. W. E. (1975): Science *190*, 529

Sondhaus C. A., Thorell B. (1960): Blood *16*, 1285

Soreq H., Nudel U., Salomon R., Revel M., Littauer U. Z. (1974): J. mol. Biol. *88*, 233

Speyer B. E., Fielding J. (1974): Biochim. biophys. Acta (Amst.) *332*, 192

Spirin A. S., Gavrilova L. P. (1969): The Ribosome. Springer Verlag New York

Spivak J. L. (1976): Blood *47*, 581

Staehelin T., Trachsel H., Erni B., Boschetti A., Schreier M. H.: Proc. 10th FEBS Meeting (in press)

Steggles A. W., Wilson G. N., Kantor J. A., Picciano D. J., Falvey A. K., Anderson W. F. (1974): Proc. nat. Acad. Sci. (Wash.) *71*, 1219

Stohlman F. Jr. (1967): Seminars Hemat. *4*, 304

Stohlman F., Jr. (1970) In: Formation and Destruction of Blood Cells. (Ed. by Greenwalt T. J. and Jamieson G. A.) J. B. Lippincot Co., Philadelphia and Toronto, p. 65

Stohlman F. Jr., Beland A., Howard D. (1963): J. clin. Invest. *42*, 984

Stohlman F. Jr., Lucarelli G., Howard D., Morse B., Leventhal B. (1969): Medicine *43*, 651

Storring P. L., Fatih S. (1975): Biochim. biophys. Acta (Amst.) *392*, 26

Sullivan A. L., Grasso J. A., Weintraub L. R. (1976): Blood *47*, 133

Sullivan A. L., Weintraub L. R. (1973): Med. Clin. North Amer. *57*, 335

Tait G. H. (1968): General aspects of haem synthesis. In: Porphyrins and Related Compounds. (Ed. by Goodwin T. W.) Academic Press, London and New York, p. 19

Takaku F., Nakao K. (1971) In: The Regulation of Erythropoiesis and Haemoglobin Synthesis. (Ed. by Trávníček T. and Neuwirt J.) Universita Karlova, Praha, p. 336

Tanaka Y. (1970): Blood *35/6*, 793

Tanaka Y., Brecher G., Bull B. (1966): Blood *28*, 758

Tavill A. S., Grayzel A. I., London I. M., Williams M. K., Vanderhoff G. A. (1968): J. biol. Chem. *243*, 4987

Taylor J. M., Dozy A., Kan Y. W., Varmus H. E., Lie-Injo L. E., Ganeson J., Todd D. (1974): Nature (Lond.) *251*, 392

Temple G. F., Housman G. E. (1972): Proc. nat. Acad. Sci. (Wash.) *69*, 1574

Terada M., Banks J., Marks P. A. (1971): J. mol. Biol. *62*, 347

Terada M., Cantor L., Metafora S., Rifkind R. A., Bank A., Marks P. A. (1972): Proc. nat. Acad. Sci. (Wash.) *69*, 3575

Terada M., Ramirez F., Cantor L., Maniatias G. M., Bank A., Rifkind R. A., Marks P. A. (1975) In: Erythropoiesis. Proceedings of the Fourth International Conference on Erythropoiesis (Ed. by Nakao K., Fisher J. W., and Takaku F.) University of Tokyo Press, p. 23

Thorell B. (1947): Acta med. Scand., Suppl. *200*, 129, 1

Trávníček T., Trávníčková E., Šulc K. (1966): Physiol. bohemoslov. *15*, 175

Trentin J. J. (1970) In: Regulation of Hematopoiesis. (Ed. by Gordon A. S.) Appleton-Century-Crofts, New York, p. 161

Tuboi S., Haysaka S. (1973): Enzyme *16*, 86

Veda K., Akedo H., Suda M. (1960): J. Biochem. (Tokyo) *48*, 584

Van Bockxmeer F., Hemmaplardh D., Morgan E. H. (1975) In: Proteins of Iron Storage and Transport in Biochemistry and Medicine (Ed. by Crichton R. R.) North-Holland Publishing Company, Amsterdam, p. 111

Van der Weyden M., Rother M., Firkin B. (1972): Brit. J. Haemat. *22*, 299

Vaquero C., Reibel L., Delaunay J., Schapira G. (1973): Biochem. biophys. Res. Commun. *54*, 1171

Vavra J. D. (1967): J. clin. Invest. *46*, 1127

Verma I. M., Temple G. F., Fan H., Baltimore D. (1972): Nature New Biol. *235*, 163

Vogler W. R., Mingioli E. S. (1965): New Engl. J. Med. *273*, 347

Von Ehrenstein G., Lipmann F. (1961): Proc. nat. Acad. Sci. (Wash.) *47*, 941

Von Ehrenstein G., Weisblum B., Benzer S. (1963): Proc. nat. Acad. Sci. (Wash.) *49*, 669

Waldman A. A., Goldstein J. (1973): Biochim. biophys. Acta (Amst.) *331*, 243

Walsh R. J., Thomas E. D., Chow S. K., Fluharty R. G., Finch C. A. (1949): Science *110*, 396

Ward H. P. (1966): J. Lab. clin. Med. *68*, 400

Warner J. R., Knopf P. M., Rich A. (1963): Proc. nat. Acad. Sci. (Wash.) *49*, 122

Warner J. R., Rich A., Hall C. E. (1962): Science *138*, 1399

Wasi P., Na-Nakor N., Pootrakul S. (1974): Clinics in Haemat. 3, 383

Watson J. D. (1970): Molecular Biology of the Gene (2nd ed.). Benjamin, New York

Waxman A. D., Collins A., Tschudy D. P. (1966): Biochem. biophys. Res. Commun. 24, 675

Waxman H. S. (1970): J. clin. Invest. 49/4, 701

Waxman H. S., Freedman M. L., Rabinovitz M. (1967): Biochem. biophys. Acta (Amst.) 145, 353

Waxman H. S., Rabinovitz M. (1965): Biochem. biophys. Res. Commun. 19, 538

Waxman H. S., Rabinovitz M. (1966): Biochim. biophys. Acta (Amst.) 129, 369

Weatherall D. J., Clegg J. B. (1972): The Thalassaemia Syndromes. Oxford University Press, Blackwell Scientific Publications Ltd. London and New York

Weatherall D. J., Clegg J. B. (1975a): Brit. J. Haemat. (Suppl.) 31, 133

Weatherall D. J., Clegg J. B. (1975b): Philos, Trans. of the Royal Soc. London B 271, 411

Weatherall D. J., Clegg J. B., Naughton M. A. (1965): Nature (Lond.) 208, 1061

Weisblum B., Cherayil J. D., Bock R. M., Söll D. (1967): J. mol. Biol. 28, 275

Weissman E. B., Cheng I. C., Orten J. M. (1973): Enzyme 16, 286

Welland F., Schwartz H. C. (1966): Clin. Res. 14, 142

White J. M., Brain M. C., Ali M. A. M. (1971): Brit. J. Haemat. 20, 263

White J. M., Harvey D. R. (1972): Nature (Lond.) 236, 71

White J. M., Hoffbrand A. U. (1974): Nature (Lond.) 248, 88

White J. M., Lang A., Lehmann H. (1972): Nature New Biol. 240, 271

Wickramasinghe S. N., Fulker M. J., Losowsky M. S. (1971): Acta Haemat. 45, 236

Wigle D. T. (1973): Europ. J. Biochem. 35, 11

Williams D. M., Loukopoulos D., Lee G. R., Cartwright G. E. (1976): Blood 48, 77

Williams S. C., Woodworth R. C. (1973): J. biol. Chem. 248, 5848

Williamson R. (1973): FEBS Letters 37, 1

Williamson R., Crossley J., Humphries S. (1974): Biochemistry 13, 703

Williamson R., Drewienkiewicz C. E., Paul J. (1973): Nature New Biol. 241, 66

Williamson R., Morrison M., Lanyon G., Eason R., Paul J. (1971): Biochemistry 10, 3014

Wilson D. B., Dintzis H. (1969): Cold Spring Harbor Symp. quant. Biol. 34, 313

Wilson D. B., Dintzis H. M. (1970): Proc. nat. Acad. Sci. (Wash.) 66, 1282

Wilson G. N., Steggles A. W., Kantor J. A., Nienhuis A. W., Anderson W. F. (1975): J. biol. Chem. 250, 8604

Winslow R. M., Ingram V. M. (1966): J. biol. Chem. 241, 1144

Winter G. C., Christensen H. N. (1965): J. biol. Chem. 240, 3594

Winterhalter K. H., Heywood J. D., Huehns E. R., Finch C. A. (1969): Brit. J. Haemat. 16, 523

Winterhalter K. H., Huehns E. R. (1963): J. clin. Invest. 42, 995

Winterhalter K. H., Huehns E. R. (1964): J. biol. Chem. 239, 3699

Wise W. C., Archdeacon J. W. (1965): Proc. Soc. exp. Biol. (N.Y.) 118/3, 653

Wise W. C., Archdeacon J. W. (1967): Experientia 23, 627

Wise W. C., Archdeacon J. W. (1969): J. gen. Physiol. 53, 487

Wolf J. L., Mason R. G., Honig G. R. (1973): Proc. nat. Acad. Sci. (Wash.) 70, 3405

Woodley C. L., Chen Y. C., Bose K. K., Gupta N. K. (1972): Biochem. biophys. Res. Commun. 46, 839

Woodward W. R., Adamson S. D., McQueen H. M., Larson J. W., Estvanik S. M., Wilairat P., Herbert E. (1973): J. biol. Chem. 248, 1556

Workman E. F., Bates G. W. (1974): Biochem. Biophys. Res. Commun. *58*, 787

Workman E. F., Bates G. W. (1975) In: Proteins of Iron Storage and Transport in Biochemistry and Medicine (Ed. by Crichton R. R.), North-Holland Publishing Company, Amsterdam, p. 155

Workman E. F., Jr., Graham G., Bates G. W. (1975): Biochim. biophys. Acta (Amst.) *399*, 254

Yamada H., Gabuzda T. G. (1974a): J. Lab. clin. Med. *83*, 478

Yamada H., Gabuzda T. G. (1974b): Blood *43*, 875

Yamada H., Hotta T., Gabuzda T. G. (1975): Proc. of the 2nd International Congress on Pathological Physiology, Prague (Abstr. No. 456)

Yang P. C., Hamada K., Scheet R. (1968): Arch. Biochem. Biophys. *125*, 506

Yannoni C. Z., Robinson S. H. (1975): Nature (Lond.) *258*, 330

Yataganas X., Gahrton G., Thorell B. (1970): Exp. Cell Res. *62*, 254

Yoneyama Y., Matsui I., Ohyama M., Yoshikawa W. (1963): Acta haemat. (Basel) *29*, 129

Yoneyama Y., Ohyama H., Sugita Y., Yoshikawa H. (1962): Biochim. biophys. Acta (Amst.) *62*, 261

Yoshida A., Lin W. (1972): J. biol. Chem. *247*, 952

Yoshida A., Watanabe S., Morris J. (1970): Proc. nat. Acad. Sci. (Wash.) *67*, 1600

Yoshikawa H., Yoneyama Y. (1964): Iron Metabolism (Ed. by Gross F.) Springer Verlag, Berlin, p. 24

Yunis A. A., Arimura G. K. (1965): J. Lab. clin. Med. *66*, 177

Zail S. C., Charleton R. W., Torrance J. D., Bothwell T. H. (1964): J. clin. Invest. *43*, 670

Zapolski E. J., Ganz R., Princiotto J. V. (1974): Amer. J. Physiol. *226*, 334

Zehavi-Willner T. (1970): Biochem. biophys. Res. Commun. *39*, 161

Zehavi-Willner T., Danon D. (1972): FEBS Letters *26*, 151

Zucker W. V., Schulman H. M. (1967): Biochim. biophys. Acta (Amst.) *138*, 400

Zucker W. V., Schulman H. M. (1968): Proc. nat. Acad. Sci. (Wash.) *59*, 582

Zuyderhoudt F. M. J., Borst P., Huijing F. (1969): Biochim. biophys. Acta (Amst.) *178*, 408

SUBJECT INDEX

Actinomycin D, 72
Acute intermittent porphyria, 71
Affinity chromatography, mRNA isolation,
  92 – 93
Alcohol, 168
Allyl-isopropylacetamide (AIA), 72
Aminoacetic acid, 64
Amino acids
  membrane transport, 50
δ- Aminolaevulinic acid (ALA)
  effect of haem synthesis, 80 – 81
  ratio NADH-NAD, 60
  role of glycine, 59
  succinyl CoA, 60
  synthesis, 59
δ- Aminolaevulinic acid (ALA) dehydratase
  inhibition by lead, 64
  purification of, 64
δ- Aminolaevulinic acid (ALA) synthetase
  activation by cystine, 61
  cytoplasmatic, 63, 77
  effect of haem on, 74
  in differentiation, 155
  limiting effect on porphyrin synthesis, 61
  mitochondrial, 63, 77
  purification of, 62
Aminomalonate, 63
Anaemia
  copper deficiency, 167
  congenital atransferrinaemia, 166
  impaired globin synthesis, 172
  iron deficiency, 163
  macrocytic, 162
  microcytic, 162, 166
  sickle-cell, 141
  sideroblastic, 167
Ascorbic acid, 67
ATP, 22, 61
ATPase, 23

Bicarbonate, 15
Bilirubin, 85
Biliverdin reductase, 85

Cell cycle, 146
Cell-free system
  chick embryo brain, 96
  from ascitic mouse cells, 95
  from liver cells, 95
  from reticulocytes, role of haem in globin
  synthesis, 130 – 132
  from wheat embryo, 95 – 96
  haemoglobin synthesis in, 91, 95 – 98,
  130 – 132
  postmicrosomal supernatant, rat liver,
  96 – 97
  postmitochondrial supernatants, 95 – 96
Centrifugation in sucrose gradient
  method for globin mRNA isolation, 91
Chelating agents, 23
  bipyridine, 45, 133
  citrate, 23
  effect on globin synthesis, 129 – 133
Chloramphenicol, 68, 168
Chromatin, see Erythroblasts
Citrate, 23
Cobalt, 72
Copper, 167
Coproporphyrinogen, 66
Corproporphyrinogen oxidase, 66
Cyclic AMP
  effect of erythropoietin on, 156
  effect on ALA synthesis, 61
  effect on HCR, 132
  effect on iron uptake, 50
Cycloheximide
  effect on level of uncommitted haem,
  137 – 139
  haem accumulation in mitochondria, 138
  inhibition of haem synthesis, 143
  inhibition of iron uptake, 39
Cycloserine, 168
Cytochrome 450, 72
Cytochrome oxidase, 167

1,4-Dihydro-2, 4, 6-trimethylpyridine
  (DDC), 70

Dimethylsulfoxide, 158
Dihydroxycoprostan, 71
2,4-Dinitrophenol, 21
Dissociation factors, 108, 122
DNA
  complementary to mRNA, 99 – 100
  effect of erythropoietin on (DNA)
  synthesis, 153
  functions in protein synthesis, 87
  transcription into mRNA, 87
DNA-DNA hybridization, 172
DNA polymerase
  inhibition by haem, 136
  RNA-dependent, 99
DNA-RNA hybridization
  method for globin mRNA detection,
  99 – 100, 104, 172

Elongation factors, 120
Emetine, 142
Endocytosis, 18
End-product inhibition, 74
Erythroblasts, 124
  basophilic, 145
  chromatin, acidic proteins from, 105
  chromatin, transcription into globin
  mRNA, 105
  control of cell division by haemoglobin,
  146
  DNA synthesis, 144
  globin mRNA isolation, 100
  HnRNA in, 104
  maturation and DNA repression, 146
  orthochromatic, 144
  polychromatophilic, 144
  regulation of maturation, 144
  RNA synthesis, 124
Erythroid cell,
  differentiation, 149
  maturation, 144
  proliferation, 161
Erythropoiesis, 149, 151, 161
Erythropoietic porphyria, 65, 82

Erythropoietin
  and sensitive phase of cell cycle, 153, 157
  as de-repressor, 105, 151, 152
  cell membrane, 153
  DNA synthesis, 153
  haem synthesis, 155
  iron uptake, 154
  mechanism of action, 151
  receptor, 156
  RNA synthesis, 152
Erythropoietin responsive cell, 105, 150
Ethacrynic acid, 23
Ethylenediaminedi-(o-hydroxyphenyl)-acetic
  acid, 23
Ethylenediaminetetracetate (EDTA)
  release of 15 s mRNP from polyribosomes,
  91, 103
Exocytosis, 19

Ferrihaemoglobin, 139
Ferritin
  apoferritin, 25
  bone marrow ferritin, 25
  haemoglobin synthesis, 26
Ferriprotoporphyrin, 74
Ferrochelatase, 66
Ferroprotoporphyrin, 74
Friend leukaemia virus, 158
Frog oocytes
  effect of haemin on mRNA translation, 132
  translation of globin mRNA in, 95, 104

Globin chain synthesis
  elongation, 119 – 120
  feedback mechanism in control of,
  127 – 129
  initiation, 113 – 118, 128
  methionyl-tRNA, role in, 113 – 115, 132
  rate limiting step, 126
  ratio of α- and β-chain synthesis, 96,
  98 – 99, 124
  regulation of, 122 – 134
  role of haem in, 129 – 134
  synchronization of, 127
  termination, 121 – 122

Globin dimer, 127, 129, 133, 139, 140
Globin genes, 123
  amplification, lack of, 123
Globin synthesis
  control of, 122 – 134
  general outline, 87 – 89
Glycine transport
  effect of haem on, 50, 84, 136
Glutathione, 67

Haem synthesis, 55
  catabolism, 85, 135
  coordination with globin synthesis,
  139 – 144
  deficiency and globin synthesis, 129
  dissociation from haemoglobin, 139
  effect on globin synthesis, 125, 129 – 134
  effect on glycine transport, 136
  endogenous pool in erythroid cells, 129,
  132, 135, 136 – 139
  feedback inhibition of haem synthesis by,
  139
  free, 86, 136 – 139
  non-haemoglobin, 136 – 138
  oxygenase, 85, 135
  regulation of, 69
  synthesis, 55
  uncommitted, 86, 136, 139
Haemsynthetase, see Ferrochelatase
Haemopoietic inductive microenviroment,
  150
Haemin
  increased globin synthesis, 129, 139
  inhibition of iron entry into reticulocytes,
  36, 45
  stimulation of globin chain initiation, 131
Haemin-controlled repressor, 131 – 134
  effect of temperature on formation of, 131,
  133
  effect on methionyl-tRNA$_f$, 132
  effect on non-haemoglobin protein
  synthesis, 132
Haemoglobin
  assembly of, 134, 139 – 140

control of erythroblast cell division, 146
  synthesis, control of, 135 – 144
Haemoglobin H disease, 173
Haemoglobin types
  Gower, 11 1, 2
  haemoglobin A, A$_2$, 11
  haemoglobin Barts, 173
  haemoglobin F, 11
  haemoglobin H, 173
Haemoglobin variants
  Constant Spring, 103, 121, 174
  Cranston, 103
  Lepore, 175
  Wayne, 103, 121
Haemosiderin, 164
N-β-Hydroxyethyl-iminodiacetic acid, 23
α-Hydroxy-haem, 85

Imidazol, 23
Ineffective erythropoiesis, 161
Initiation codon, 103, 113
Initiation factors, 95, 98, 108, 117 – 118, 131
INH, see Isonicotinic acid hydrazide,
Iron
  bivalent, 67
  complexes, 26
  cytosol iron, 26
  ferritin iron, 25
  haemoglobin synthesis, 34
  intracellular kinetics, 24
  mitochondrial, 27
  non-haem, 26
  supply to erythroid cells, 15
  transferrin iron, 16, 20
  trivalent, 67, 84
Iron uptake, 14, 20, 23
  effect of haem, 36, 45, 142
  inhibition of globin synthesis, 38
  inhibitors of haem synthesis, 38
  sideroblastic anaemia, 170
Isonicotinic acid hydrazide, 29, 37, 40, 79
  effect on globin synthesis, 129, 130, 133

Krebs cycle, 84

Lead
  effect on globin synthesis, 129
  effect on haem synthesis, 64, 68, 85
  effect on iron incorporation, 29
  sideroblastic anaemias, 168

Messenger RNA, *see* RNA
Microcytosis, 162
Microsomal haemoprotein, 72
Mitochondria
  haem accumulation after cycloheximide, 138
  role in iron metabolism, 27
  site of haem production, 57, 135, 136, 139
Mitosis, 146, 162
Molecular hybridization, *see* DNA-RNA hybridization

NAD, 60
NADH, 22, 60
Nitrilotriacetic acid, 23
Nucleohistone, 146

Oligomycin, 21
O-Methyl-threonine
  α- and β-globin mRNA isolation, 93
  inhibition of globin chain synthesis, 111, 128
  mRNA stability, 125
Ouabain, 23
δ-Oximinolaevulinic acid, 64

Penicillamine, 42, 80
Phenol extraction
  mRNA isolation, 92
Phosphodiesterase, 22
Phosphatidylic acid, 67
Phospholipase A, 67
Pinocytosis, 16
Poly(A)-Sepharose affinity chromatography
  mRNA isolation, 92
Porphobilinogen, 64
  isomerase, 64
Porphobilinogen oxygenase, 85

Proerythroblasts, 144
  induction of globin mRNA, 152
Protoporphyrin, 66
  free, 68
  in iron deficiency, 167
Protoporphyrinogen, 66
Puromycin
  effect on iron uptake, 39
  release of 20 s mRNP from polyribosomes, 91
Pyrazinamide, 168
Pyridoxal kinase, 168
Pyridoxal phosphate, 40
Pyridoxal phosphate phosphatase, 168
Pyrrolinone, 85

Release factors, 121
Reticulocytes
  cytoplasmatic control of globin synthesis, 124 – 134
  globin mRNA isolation, 90
  haem pool in. 129, 136 – 139
  maturation, haemoglobin synthesis, 140
  membrane, 17
  microtubules, 18
  mitochondria, 27, 33, 57
  rabbit, α- and β-globin mRNA content, 98
  ribosomes, 89
  transferrin receptors, 17
Reticuloendothelial cells, 15, 167
Reverse transcriptase, *see* DNA polymerase, RNA-dependent
Rhodopseudomonas spheroides, 61
Ribonuclease, 110
  in nucleated erythroid cells, 100, 125
Ribosomal RNA, *see* RNA
Ribosomes
  acceptor site, 120
  dissociation into sub-units, 91, 110, 122
  donor site, 120
  for α- and β-chains, 128
  globin synthesis, role in, 107
  membrane-bound, 112
  polyribosome disaggregation, 111

204

polyribosomes, 110, 120, 135
proteins in, 108
ribosomal sub-units, 95, 98, 109, 111, 118, 122
RNA in, *see* RNA, ribosomal

RNA
biosynthesis of, 89, 104 – 106, 159, 160
characteristics of, 100 – 104
codons for amino acids, 88
detection of, 95 – 100
effect of erythropoietin on formation of, 152
electron microscopy, 105
functions in haemoglobin synthesis, 89, 95 – 98, 107, 109 – 122
gene expression, control of, 105, 123
haem, role in transcription, 105
haemin, effect on initiation, 103 – 132
heterogenous nuclear (HnRNA), 104, 124
in post-ribosomal supernatant, 93 – 94, 104
isolation of, 91 – 94, 100
lack of synthesis in reticulocytes, 89, 124
messenger for globin, 89
methylated constituents, 103
molecular structure of, 101 – 103
nuclear events, 104, 124
poly(A) sequence in, 99, 100 – 103, 105, 124
pre-messenger, 104, 105
protein synthesis, general outline of, 87 – 89
ribosomal, 89, 109
separation of α- and β-globin messenger, 93, 94, 100
stability, 124
transcription of DNA into, 104 – 106, 123
transfer, 89, 95, 98, 106 – 107, 117, 119, 120, 126
translation of, 95 – 99, 125, 128
transport from nucleus, 105
untranslated sequences of, 101 – 103
RNA polymerase
DNA-dependent, 105
effect of erythropoietin, 153

inhibition by haem, 136, 148
RNA-dependent, 106, 148
RNA replicase, *see* RNA polymerase, RNA-dependent
Rropheocytosis, 15
Rotenone, 21

Sideroblastic anaemia
hereditary form, 170
primary acquired, 170
secondary, 170
Sideroblasts, 164
Siderochelin, 27
Sideroglobin, 26
Sodium dodecyl sulphate (SDS)
release of 9 s mRNA from polyribosomes, 91
Stem cell, 150
erythroid committed, 105, 150
Steroid
dehydroepiandrosterone, 70
erythroid differentiation, 150
ethiocholanone, 70
5-β-H steroids, 70
Succinate, 60, 84
Succinyl-CoA, 55, 59, 84
Succinyl-CoA synthetase, 60
Sulfhydryl groups, 22

Termination codons, 121, 174
Thalassaemia
accumulation of globin chains, 128
haemoglobin Constant Spring, 174
haemoglobin Lepore, 175
proteolytic enzymes, 135
α-thalassaemia, 173
β- and δ_3-thalassaemias, 174
Transfer RNA, *see* RNA
Translocase, *see* Elongation factors
Transpeptidase, 120
Trihydroxycoprostan, 71
Transferrin
apotransferrin, 20
atransferrinaemia, 166

binding sites, 21
iron release from, 22, 48
receptors, 17
saturation, 20

Uroporphyrinogen III, 63
    cosynthetase, 64
Uroporphyrinogen decarboxylase, 66
Uroporphyrinogen I
    synthetase, 64

Wheat embryo cell-free system
    translation of globin mRNA in, 95 – 96